CONGRESSIONAL POLICIES, PRACTICES AND PROCEDURES

KEY CONGRESSIONAL REPORTS FOR JUNE 2019

HEALTH

CONGRESSIONAL POLICIES, PRACTICES AND PROCEDURES

Additional books and e-books in this series can be found on Nova's website under the Series tab.

CONGRESSIONAL POLICIES, PRACTICES AND PROCEDURES

KEY CONGRESSIONAL REPORTS FOR JUNE 2019

HEALTH

AMADA A. BYRD
EDITOR

snova
New York

NOTICE TO THE READER

Additional color graphics may be available in the e-book version of this book.

Library of Congress Cataloging-in-Publication Data

ISBN: 978-1-53616-665-1

Published by Nova Science Publishers, Inc. † New York

CONTENTS

PREFACE

This book is a comprehensive compilation of all reports, testimony, correspondence and other publications issued by the Congressional Research Service on Health during the month of June.

Chapter 1 - When the Food and Drug Administration (FDA) approves a drug for sale in the United States, the approval includes a section entitled "Indications for Use." This section lists the one or more diseases, conditions, or symptoms for which the drug's sponsor (usually the manufacturer) has provided, to FDA's satisfaction, evidence in support of the drug's safety and effectiveness. FDA approval is also based on its review of the drug's dosage, packaging, manufacturing plan, and labeling. Before changing any of those elements, the sponsor must inform, and usually receive permission from, FDA. In essence, FDA regulates all approval and post-approval aspects of a drug product. But FDA traditionally has not regulated the practice of medicine. Physicians, therefore, may prescribe an FDA-approved drug for indications that FDA has not reviewed for safety and effectiveness. Those uses, furthermore, are not addressed in the labeling information regarding, among other things, dosing, warnings about interactions with other drugs, and possible adverse events. *How Are Off-Label Prescription Drugs Used?* Prescribing for so-called off-label uses can be accepted medical practice, often reflecting cutting-edge clinical expertise. For example, this is the case with oncology drug use, more than half of which is off-label. Off-label prescribing can be a reasonable choice when labeling overlooks certain populations—for example, when a drug tested in adults is prescribed to children. A drug may be used off-label when it was tested for the treatment of one disease and prescribed in an attempt to prevent or treat another, when it was tested at one dose and used at higher or lower doses, or when it was tested in an eight-week trial and prescribed for long-term use. Estimates for how common off-label prescriptions are in the United States are hardly precise. Credible researchers have estimated they make up as little as 12% and as much as 38% of doctor-office prescriptions. *What Are the Risks of Off-Label Prescriptions?* Prescriptions for off-label uses of FDA-approved drugs are made without the benefit of an FDA-reviewed analysis of safety and effectiveness data. Physicians may resort to such prescribing to take advantage of new ideas and treatment approaches when available information to support them is inadequate. However, despite the potential risks associated with off-label uses, efforts to prohibit such uses might hurt the public. Some off-label prescribing may result because manufacturers have chosen not to invest the resources needed to have FDA add indications to the drug's approval and labeling. A worst-case scenario for the nation's health would be the widespread acceptance of a drug for an off-label use that sufficient research would have revealed to be ineffective, unsafe, or both. Aside from the drug's direct harm, the time spent waiting to see whether it worked would have been time not spent exploring other treatment options. Unchecked off-label prescribing may also threaten the FDA gold standard of drug approval. If clinicians had already accepted a new use into practice through off-label prescribing, a manufacturer may choose to not invest resources to go through clinical trials and the FDA process to win approval. Although manufacturers do share information on off-label uses, courts have sometimes found they had overstepped allowable bounds. Congress has given permission for limited sharing. Are there other ways to share clinical information that do not put the public's health or FDA's authority at risk? *What Role Can Congress Play in the Use of Off-Label Prescriptions?* How might Congress, in its legislative or oversight roles, consider the use of off-label drugs to protect the public's health? Legislators and health analysts have suggested both restrictive and permissive actions regarding off-label use. Ideas—some of which conflict with others—include

- disclosure to patients;
- data collection, availability, and analysis;
- dissemination of clinical data;
- linking reimbursement and coverage to evidence of safety and effectiveness;
- clinical research and research transparency;
- clinical guidance;
- congressional oversight through the Government Accountability Office, the Federal Trade Commission, and the Department of Health and Human Services; and
- consideration of other countries' approaches to off-label use.

Some actions would require federal legislation. Other proposals would involve actions by other entities, such as state authorities and professional organizations, which Congress could urge.

Chapter 2 - Medicaid is a means-tested entitlement program that finances the delivery of primary and acute medical services as well as long-term services and supports (LTSS) to an estimated 75 million people at a cost to states and the federal government of $616 billion in FY2018. Medicaid is one of the largest payers in the U.S. health care system, representing 17% of national health care spending in CY2017; in that year, private health insurance and Medicare accounted for 34% and 20% of national health care spending, respectively. Participation in Medicaid is voluntary for states, though all states, the District of Columbia, and the territories choose to participate. The federal government requires states to cover certain mandatory populations and services, but the federal government also allows states to cover other optional populations and services. Due to this flexibility, there is substantial variation among the states in terms of factors such as Medicaid eligibility, covered benefits, and provider payment rates. Historically, Medicaid eligibility generally has been limited to low-income children, pregnant women, parents of dependent children, the elderly, and individuals with disabilities; however, since 2014, states have had the option to cover nonelderly adults with income up to 133% of the federal poverty level (FPL) under the Patient Protection and Affordable Care Act (ACA; P.L. 111- 148, as amended) Medicaid expansion. Medicaid coverage includes a variety of primary and acute-care services as well as LTSS. Not all Medicaid enrollees have access to the same set of services. An enrollee's eligibility pathway determines the available services within a benefit package. Federal law provides two primary benefit packages for state Medicaid programs: (1) traditional benefits and (2) alternative benefit plans (ABPs). Beneficiary cost sharing (e.g., premiums and co-payments) is limited under the Medicaid program. Medicaid enrollees generally receive benefits via one of two service delivery systems: fee-forservice (FFS) or managed care. Under FFS, health care providers are paid by the state Medicaid program for each service provided to a Medicaid enrollee. Under managed care, Medicaid enrollees get most or all of their services through an organization under contract with the state. Most states use a combination of FFS and managed care. The federal government and the states jointly finance Medicaid. The federal government reimburses states for a portion of each state's Medicaid program costs. Federal Medicaid funding is an open-ended entitlement to states, which means there is no upper limit or cap on the amount of federal Medicaid funds a state may receive. The Social Security Act authorizes several waiver and demonstration authorities that allow states to operate their Medicaid programs outside of federal rules. The primary Medicaid waiver authorities include Section 1115, Section 1915(b), and Section 1915(c). Medicaid provider payment rates are set by states within federal rules. In some cases, states make supplemental payments to Medicaid providers that are separate from, and in addition to, the payment rates for services rendered to Medicaid enrollees. Also, Medicaid program integrity initiatives are designed to combat fraud, waste, and abuse in the Medicaid program.

Chapter 3 - This chapter describes selected health care-related provisions that are scheduled to expire during the first session of the116th

Congress (i.e., during calendar year [CY] 2019). For purposes of this chapter, *expiring provisions* are defined as portions of law that are time-limited and will lapse once a statutory deadline is reached absent further legislative action. The expiring provisions included in this chapter are those related to Medicare, Medicaid, State Children's Health Insurance Program (CHIP), and private health insurance programs and activities. The report also includes health care-related provisions that were enacted in the Patient Protection and Affordable Care Act (ACA; P.L. 111-148) or last extended under the Bipartisan Budget Act of 2018 (BBA 2018; P.L. 115-123). In addition, this chapter describes health care-related provisions within the same scope that expired during the 115th Congress (i.e., during CY2017 or CY2018). This chapter generally focuses on two types of health care-related provisions within the scope discussed above. The first type of provision provides or controls mandatory spending, meaning that it provides temporary funding, temporary increases or decreases in funding (e.g., Medicare provider bonus payments), or temporary special protections that may result in changes in funding levels (e.g., Medicare funding provisions that establish a floor). The second type of provision defines the authority of government agencies or other entities to act, usually by authorizing a policy, project, or activity. Such provisions also may temporarily delay the implementation of a regulation, requirement, or deadline, or establish a moratorium on a particular activity. Expiring health care provisions that are predominantly associated with discretionary spending activities—such as discretionary authorizations of appropriations and authorities for discretionary user fees—are excluded from this report. Certain types of provisions with expiration dates that otherwise would meet the criteria set forth above are excluded from this chapter. Some of these provisions are excluded because they are transitional or routine in nature or have been superseded by congressional action that otherwise modifies the intent of the expiring provision. For example, statutorily required Medicare payment rate reductions and payment rate re-basings that are implemented over a specified time period are not considered to require legislative attention and are excluded. The chapter provides tables listing the relevant provisions that are scheduled to expire in 2019 and that expired in 2018 or 2017. The chapter then describes each listed provision, including a legislative history. An appendix lists relevant demonstration projects and pilot programs that are scheduled to expire in 2019 or that expired in 2018 or 2017. This chapter describes selected health care-related provisions that are scheduled to expire during the first session of the 116th Congress (i.e., during calendar year [CY] 2019). For purposes of this chapter, *expiring provisions* are defined as portions of law that are time-limited and will lapse once a statutory deadline is reached, absent further legislative action. The expiring provisions included in this chapter are those related to Medicare, Medicaid, State Children's Health Insurance Program (CHIP), and private health insurance programs and activities. The report also includes health care-related provisions that were enacted in the Patient Protection and Affordable Care Act (ACA; P.L. 111-148) or last extended under the Bipartisan Budget Act of 2018 (BBA 2018; P.L. 115-123). In addition, this chapter describes health care-related provisions within the same scope that expired during the 115th Congress (i.e., during CY2017 or CY2018).. This chapter generally focuses on two types of health care-related provisions within the scope discussed above. The first type of provision provides or controls mandatory spending, meaning that it provides temporary funding, temporary increases or decreases in funding (e.g., Medicare provider bonus payments), or temporary special protections that may result in changes in funding levels (e.g., Medicare funding provisions that establish a floor). Mandatory spending is controlled by authorization acts; discretionary spending is controlled by appropriations acts. The second type of provision defines the authority of government agencies or other entities to act, usually by authorizing a policy, project, or activity. Such provisions also may temporarily delay the implementation of a regulation, requirement, or deadline, or establish a moratorium on a particular activity. Expiring health care provisions that are predominantly associated with discretionary spending activities—such as discretionary authorizations of appropriations and authorities for discretionary user fees—are excluded from this chapter. Certain types of provisions with expiration dates that otherwise would meet the criteria set forth above are excluded from this chapter. Some of these provisions are excluded because they are transitional or routine in nature or have been superseded by congressional action that otherwise modifies the intent of the expiring provision. For example, statutorily required Medicare payment rate reductions and payment rate re-basings that are implemented over a specified time period are not considered to require legislative attention and are excluded. The report is organized as follows: Table 1 lists the relevant provisions that are scheduled to expire in 2019. Table 2 lists the relevant provisions that expired during 2018 or 2017. The provisions in each table are organized by expiration date and applicable health care-related program. The report then describes each listed provision, including a legislative history. The summaries are grouped by provisions that are scheduled to expire in 2019 followed by those that expired in 2018 or 2017.[1] Appendix A lists demonstration projects and pilot programs that are scheduled to expire in 2019 or that expired in 2018 or 2017 and are related to Medicare, Medicaid, CHIP, and private health insurance programs and activities or other health care-related provisions that were enacted in the ACA or last extended under the BBA 2018. Appendix B lists all laws that created, modified, or extended the health care-related expiring provisions described in this chapter. Appendix C lists abbreviations used in the report.

Chapter 4 - The substantial burden of opioid abuse related to the current opioid epidemic in the United States has resulted in a disparity between the need for substance abuse treatment and the current capacity. Methadone and buprenorphine are two medications used in medication-assisted treatment (MAT) for opioid use disorder (OUD). Methadone and buprenorphine are both opioids; their use to treat opioid use disorders is often called *opioid agonist treatment* or *therapy* (OAT) or *opioid agonist MAT*. As controlled substances, methadone and buprenorphine are subject to additional regulations. Methadone may be used to treat opioid addiction within federally certified opioid treatment programs (OTP)—often referred to as methadone clinics. Buprenorphine may be used to treat opioid use

[1] The 2019 expiring provisions are further organized by Social Security Act (SSA) and Public Health Service Act (PHSA) title and section. A third category includes provisions that are freestanding (i.e., new laws).

disorder in two settings: (1) within an OTP and (2) outside an OTP pursuant to a Drug Addiction Treatment Act (DATA) waiver. The federal government has taken steps to increase the availability of MAT in response to the escalation of opioid overdoses and deaths in recent years. Policy efforts to address the opioid epidemic have corresponded with increased treatment availability, yet access to substance abuse treatment has not kept pace with the increasing rates of opioid addiction in the United States. Geographic information is important in accurately evaluating treatment capacity. Treatment location may be especially relevant to understanding the discrepancy between need and capacity. The current report identifies the geographic location of MAT providers using methadone and buprenorphine (opioid agonist treatment) in the United States. The analysis uses Substance Abuse and Mental Health Services Administration (SAMHSA) data to identify the number and location of (1) federally certified opioid treatment programs and (2) practitioners with DATA waivers. The geographic location of OTPs and DATA-waived practitioners are displayed in several national and regional maps. Identifying the location of OAT providers may have utility in increasing accessibility to treatment. However, simply increasing capacity for treatment may not effectively increase availability (or decrease opioid-related overdoses) if treatment providers are not located in areas of need. The current analysis does not evaluate need—by locating opioid-related overdose hospital admissions and deaths for instance. It does, however, provide an initial step in assessing how treatment providers are dispersed geographically. Other factors, such as substance use treatment financing, stigma, and waiting periods for services may also affect OAT availability. Practitioners are subject to state laws and regulations regarding prescribing privileges which affect their eligibility for DATA waivers and, in turn, the availability of treatment. Congress may incorporate geographic factors in strategies designed to increase capacity and availability of treatment.

Chapter 5 - Over the last several years, lawmakers in the United States have responded to rising drug overdose deaths, which increased four-fold from 1999 to 2017, with a variety of legislation, hearings, and oversight activities. In 2017, more than 70,000 people died from drug overdoses, and approximately 68% of those deaths involved an opioid. Many federal agencies are involved in domestic and foreign efforts to combat opioid abuse and the continuing increase in opioid related overdose deaths. A subset of those agencies confront the supply side (some may also confront the demand side) of the opioid epidemic. The primary federal agency involved in drug enforcement, including prescription opioids diversion control, is the Drug Enforcement Administration (DEA). Other federal agencies that address the illicit opioid supply include, but are not limited to, the Federal Bureau of Investigation, Offices of the U.S. Attorneys, Office of Justice Programs, U.S. Customs and Border Protection, U.S. Department of State, U.S. Postal Inspection Service, and Office of National Drug Control Policy. This chapter focuses on efforts from these departments and agencies only. Lawmakers have addressed opioid abuse as both a public health and a criminal justice issue, and Congress enacted several new laws in the 114th and 115th Congresses. These include the Comprehensive Addiction and Recovery Act of 2016 (CARA; P.L. 114-198), the 21st Century Cures Act (Cures Act; P.L. 114-255), and most recently the SUPPORT for Patients and Communities Act (SUPPORT Act; P.L. 115-271). Congress also provided funds specifically to address the opioid epidemic in FY2017-FY2019 appropriations. This chapter answers common supply and criminal justice-related questions that have arisen as drug overdose deaths in the United States continue to increase. It does *not* provide a comprehensive overview of opioid abuse as a criminal justice issue. The report is divided into the following sections:

Overview of the Opioid Epidemic in the United States;

- Overview of the Opioid Supply;
- Opioids and Domestic Supply Control Policy;
- Opioids and Foreign Supply Control Policy;
- Recent Congressional Action on the Opioid Epidemic; and
- The Opioid Epidemic and State Criminal Justice Policies.

Over the last several years, the public and lawmakers in the United States have been alarmed over the increasing number of drug overdose deaths, most of which have involved opioids. Congress has responded to the issue through legislative activity, oversight, and funding, while the Administration has sought to reduce the supply and demand of illicit drugs through enforcement, prevention, and treatment. This FAQ report answers questions about the opioid epidemic and federal efforts to control the supply of opioids. It does not provide a comprehensive overview of opioid abuse and the criminal justice response. Instead, it answers common questions that have arisen due to rising drug overdose deaths and the availability of illicit opioids in the United States.

Chapter 6 - Social Security's receipts and expenditures are accounted for through two federal trust funds: the Federal Old-Age and Survivors Insurance (OASI) Trust Fund and the Federal Disability Insurance (DI) Trust Fund. Under their intermediate assumptions and under current law, the Social Security trustees project that the DI trust fund will become depleted in 2052 and the OASI trust fund will become depleted in 2034. Although the two funds are legally separate, they are often considered in combination. The trustees project that the combined Social Security trust funds will become depleted in 2035. At that point, the combined trust funds would become *insolvent*, because incoming tax revenue would be sufficient to pay only about 80% of scheduled benefits. If a trust fund became depleted and current receipts were insufficient to cover current expenditures, there would be a conflict between two federal laws. Under the Social Security Act, beneficiaries would still be legally entitled to their full scheduled benefits. However, the Antideficiency Act prohibits government spending in excess of available funds, so the Social Security Administration (SSA) would not have legal authority to pay full Social Security benefits on time. It is unclear what specific actions SSA would take if a trust fund were insolvent. After depletion, the trust funds would continue to receive tax revenues, from which a majority of scheduled benefits could be paid. One option would be to pay full benefits on a delayed schedule; another would be to make timely but reduced payments. Social Security beneficiaries would remain legally entitled to full, timely benefits and could take legal action to claim the balance of their benefits. Maintaining financial balance after trust fund insolvency would require substantial reductions in Social Security benefits, substantial increases in tax revenues, or some combination of the two. The trustees project that following depletion of the combined funds in 2035, Congress could restore balance by reducing scheduled benefits by about 20%; the required reduction would grow gradually to 25% by 2093. An alternative could be for Congress to raise the Social Security payroll tax rate from 12.4% to 15.60% following depletion in 2035, then gradually increase it to 16.50% by 2093. Trust-fund insolvency could be avoided if expenditures were reduced or receipts increased sufficiently. The sooner Congress acts to adjust Social Security policy, the less abrupt the changes would need to be, because they could be spread over a longer period and would therefore affect a larger number of workers and beneficiaries. Even if changes were not implemented immediately, enacting them sooner would give workers and beneficiaries more time to plan and adjust their work and savings behavior.

Chapter 7 - The Radiation Exposure Compensation Act (RECA) provides one-time benefit payments to persons who may have developed cancer or other specified diseases after being exposed to radiation from atomic weapons testing or uranium mining, milling, or transporting. Administered by the Department of Justice (DOJ), RECA has awarded over $2.3 billion in benefits to more than 35,000 claimants since its inception in 1990. The RECA program is scheduled to sunset in 2022.

RECA benefits are available to the following groups:

- onsite participants—$75,000 to persons who participated onsite in the atmospheric test of an atomic weapon and developed one of the types of cancers specified in the statute;
- downwinders—$50,000 to persons who were present in one of the specified areas near the Nevada Test Site during a period of atmospheric atomic weapons testing and developed one of the types of cancers specified in the statute; and
- uranium miners, millers, and ore transporters—$100,000 to persons who worked in mining, milling, or transportation of

uranium between 1942 and 1971 and developed one of the types of diseases specified in the statute.

The RECA statute was last amended in 2000. Since then, Congress has frequently considered legislation to expand the downwinder-eligibility area by making persons who were affected in other states during periods of atmospheric atomic weapons testing eligible for benefits and by allowing uranium miners, millers, and ore transporters to qualify for benefits based on work after 1971. However, an expansion of the downwinder-eligibility area is not supported by a congressionally mandated National Research Council report on atomic test fallout, and the inclusion of post-1971 uranium work, which was largely for commercial rather than governmental purposes, is not consistent with the program's stated intent.

In: Key Congressional Reports for June 2019 ISBN: 978-1-53616-665-1
Editor: Amada A. Byrd

Chapter 1

OFF-LABEL USE OF PRESCRIPTION DRUGS*

Susan Thaul

SUMMARY

When the Food and Drug Administration (FDA) approves a drug for sale in the United States, the approval includes a section entitled "Indications for Use." This section lists the one or more diseases, conditions, or symptoms for which the drug's sponsor (usually the manufacturer) has provided, to FDA's satisfaction, evidence in support of the drug's safety and effectiveness. FDA approval is also based on its review of the drug's dosage, packaging, manufacturing plan, and labeling. Before changing any of those elements, the sponsor must inform, and usually receive permission from, FDA.

In essence, FDA regulates all approval and post-approval aspects of a drug product. But FDA traditionally has not regulated the practice of medicine. Physicians, therefore, may prescribe an FDA-approved drug for indications that FDA has not reviewed for safety and effectiveness. Those uses, furthermore, are not addressed in the labeling information regarding, among other things, dosing, warnings about interactions with other drugs, and possible adverse events.

---

* This is an edited, reformatted and augmented version of Congressional Research Service Publication No. R45792, dated July 1, 2019.

How Are Off-Label Prescription Drugs Used?

Prescribing for so-called off-label uses can be accepted medical practice, often reflecting cutting-edge clinical expertise. For example, this is the case with oncology drug use, more than half of which is off-label. Off-label prescribing can be a reasonable choice when labeling overlooks certain populations—for example, when a drug tested in adults is prescribed to children. A drug may be used off-label when it was tested for the treatment of one disease and prescribed in an attempt to prevent or treat another, when it was tested at one dose and used at higher or lower doses, or when it was tested in an eight-week trial and prescribed for long-term use. Estimates for how common off-label prescriptions are in the United States are hardly precise. Credible researchers have estimated they make up as little as 12% and as much as 38% of doctor-office prescriptions.

What Are the Risks of Off-Label Prescriptions?

Prescriptions for off-label uses of FDA-approved drugs are made without the benefit of an FDA-reviewed analysis of safety and effectiveness data. Physicians may resort to such prescribing to take advantage of new ideas and treatment approaches when available information to support them is inadequate. However, despite the potential risks associated with off-label uses, efforts to prohibit such uses might hurt the public. Some off-label prescribing may result because manufacturers have chosen not to invest the resources needed to have FDA add indications to the drug's approval and labeling.

A worst-case scenario for the nation's health would be the widespread acceptance of a drug for an off-label use that sufficient research would have revealed to be ineffective, unsafe, or both. Aside from the drug's direct harm, the time spent waiting to see whether it worked would have been time not spent exploring other treatment options.

Unchecked off-label prescribing may also threaten the FDA gold standard of drug approval. If clinicians had already accepted a new use into practice through off-label prescribing, a manufacturer may choose to not invest resources to go through clinical trials and the FDA process to win approval.

Although manufacturers do share information on off-label uses, courts have sometimes found they had overstepped allowable bounds. Congress has given permission for limited sharing. Are there other ways to share clinical information that do not put the public's health or FDA's authority at risk?

What Role Can Congress Play in the Use of Off-Label Prescriptions?

How might Congress, in its legislative or oversight roles, consider the use of off-label drugs to protect the public's health? Legislators and health analysts have suggested both restrictive and permissive actions regarding off-label use. Ideas—some of which conflict with others—include

- disclosure to patients;
- data collection, availability, and analysis;
- dissemination of clinical data;
- linking reimbursement and coverage to evidence of safety and effectiveness;
- clinical research and research transparency;
- clinical guidance;
- congressional oversight through the Government Accountability Office, the Federal Trade Commission, and the Department of Health and Human Services; and
- consideration of other countries' approaches to off-label use.

Some actions would require federal legislation. Other proposals would involve actions by other entities, such as state authorities and professional organizations, which Congress could urge.

INTRODUCTION

Both legislators and regulators have expressed concern about the safety and effectiveness of prescription drugs prescribed for "off-label uses"—purposes other than those for which the Food and Drug Administration (FDA) has approved their sale.[1] Two recent incidents illustrate the bases for those concerns.

---

[1] FDA Memorandum, "Public Health Interests and First Amendment Considerations Related to Manufacturer Communications Regarding Unapproved Uses of Approved or Cleared Medical Products" January 2017, https://www.regulations.gov/document?D=FDA-2016-N-1149-0040. See *Table A-1* for selected history of congressional concerns.

The first involves a drug already on the market. Safety experts raised concerns about ketamine, a drug available as an injectable anesthetic.[2] They noted that physicians have created outpatient clinics to administer intravenous ketamine in an off-label use to treat depression and migraines.[3] FDA has not reviewed clinical data that could support the clinics' promotional claims of safety and effectiveness.[4]

In August 2018, a second incident occurred in a Texas courtroom. Astra Zeneca settled a case concerning its alleged promotion of Seroquel for uses other than those for which it had sought and obtained FDA approval for sale in the United States.[5] The core of the complaint by the state of Texas was that the company promoted the drug's use in children, although the FDA-approved labeling of the drug was for adult use. It was one of a number of settlements since 2000 resulting in payments by drug companies for the promotion of off-label uses.[6]

To help understand the issues involving off-label use, and how these issues might concern Congress, this chapter addresses five questions:

---

[2] Megan Thielking, "A STAT Investigation: Ketamine gives hope to patients with severe depression. But some clinics stray from the science and hype its benefits," STAT, September 24, 2018, https://www.statnews.com/2018/09/24/ketamine-clinics-severe-depression-treatment; and Melvyn W. Zhang, Keith M. Harris, and Roger C. Ho, "Is Off-label repeat prescription of ketamine as a rapid antidepressant safe? Controversies, ethical concerns, and legal implications," BMC Medical Ethics, vol. 17, no. 4, published online January 14, 2016, https://www.ncbi.nlm.nih.gov/pmc/articles/PMC4714497/pdf/12910_2016_Article_87.pdf.

[3] See, for example, Actify Neurotherapies, https://www.fda.gov/downloads/AdvisoryCommittees/CommitteesMeetingMaterials/Drugs/PsychopharmacologicDrugsAdvisoryCommittee/UCM631429.pdf.

[4] In March 2019, FDA approved a new drug application for *intranasal* esketamine for treatment-resistant depression (FDA, "FDA approves new nasal spray medication for treatment-resistant depression; available only at a certified doctor's office or clinic," News Release, March 5, 2019, https://www.fda.gov/NewsEvents/Newsroom/PressAnnouncements/wucm632761.htm?dom=prime&src=syn).

[5] Ken Paxton, Attorney General of Texas, "AG Paxton Recovers $110 Million for Texas in Medicaid Fraud Settlements," News Release, August 7, 2018, https://www.texasattorneygeneral.gov/news/releases/ag-paxton-recovers110-million-texas-medicaid-fraud-settlements; https://www.texasattorneygeneral.gov/sites/default/files/files/epress/Seroquel_SA_Fully_Executed.pdf.

[6] For example, Department of Justice, "GlaxoSmithKline to Plead Guilty and Pay $3 Billion to Resolve Fraud Allegations and Failure to Report Safety Data," Office of Public Affairs, July 2, 2012, https://www.justice.gov/opa/pr/glaxosmithkline-plead-guilty-and-pay-3-billion-resolve-fraud-allegations-and-failure-report; and Department of Justice, "Fact Sheet: Significant False Claims Act Settlements & Judgments, Fiscal Years 2009-2016," https://www.justice.gov/ opa/press-release/file/918366/download.

- What is drug labeling? What is off-label use?
- How are off-label prescriptions used in medicine today?
- What are the risks and benefits associated with off-label prescriptions?
- What concerns, if any, does Congress have about such prescriptions?
- If Congress wanted to do something about off-label prescriptions, what would be some of the options?

DRUG LABELING AND OFF-LABEL USE

To market a prescription drug in the United States, a manufacturer needs FDA approval.[7] To obtain that approval, the manufacturer must demonstrate the drug's safety and effectiveness according to criteria specified in law and agency regulations. It must also ensure that its manufacturing plant passes FDA inspection.

Finally, it must obtain FDA approval for the drug's labeling—a term that covers all written material about the drug, including, for example, packaging, prescribing information for physicians, and patient brochures. FDA, thus, approves the drug and its labeling for a specific use. That use specifies the disease or condition, the population, and the way the drug is packaged and administered.

When a physician prescribes a drug for reasons other than those specified in the FDA approval and labeling, the medical profession considers this to be *off-label use*.

---

[7] FDA-approved drugs are designated by law into only two categories: prescription and nonprescription (also referred to as over-the-counter). No drug was prescription-only until the 1951 Humphrey-Durham amendments [P.L. 82-215, the Food, Drug, and Cosmetics Act Amendments Act, 1951], which stated, "A drug intended for use by man which ... because of its toxicity or other potentiality for harmful effect, or the method of its use, or the collateral measures necessary to its use, is not safe for use except under the supervision of a practitioner licensed by law to administer such drug" (FFDCA §503(b)(1)). See CRS In Focus IF10463, *Regulation of Over-the-Counter (OTC) Drugs*.

FDA regulates the drug and the manufacturer. Each state regulates clinicians and pharmacies.[8] A licensed physician may—except in highly restricted circumstances[9]—prescribe the approved drug without limitation. A prescription to an individual whose demographic or medical characteristics differ from those indicated in a drug's FDA-approved labeling is accepted medical practice.

In a 2006 study of drug prescribing by office-based physicians, 21% of prescriptions were written for off-label uses. Of those off-label prescriptions, the study's authors found that 27% were backed by strong scientific support.[10] A 2016 Canadian study of primary care clinics found an overall rate of 12% of prescriptions for off-label uses. The percentage varied, however, by therapeutic class, ranging from 5% for ear, nose, and throat medications to 25% for central nervous system medications.[11] An econometric model from the National Ambulatory Medical Care Survey estimated a 38% rate of off-label use.[12]

Research has shown that more than half of oncology drug use is off-label. A 2018 study examined 43 FDA-approved cancer drugs and compared their 99 labeled uses with the acceptable uses published by a national compendium Medicare relies on to make coverage decisions.[13] Of

---

[8] The FFDCA does not give FDA authority to regulate the practice of medicine; that responsibility generally rests with the states and medical professional associations.

[9] FDA may place restrictions on prescribing or dispensing as "elements to assure safe use" (ETASU) as part of a risk evaluation and mitigation strategy (REMS) that the agency may require (see FFDCA §505-1(f)).

[10] David C. Radley, Stan N. Finkelstein, and Randall S. Stafford, "Off-label Prescribing Among Office-Based Physicians," Archives of Internal Medicine, vol. 166, May 8, 2006. The authors note, "[a]n indication was considered to be scientifically supported if, according to DRUGDEX, its effectiveness has been shown in controlled trials or observed in clinical settings."

[11] Tewodros Eguale, David L. Buckeridge, Aman Verma, Nancy E. Winslade, Andrea Benedetti, James A. Hanley, Robyn Tamblyn, "Association of Off-label Drug Use and Adverse Drug Events in an Adult Population," *JAMA Internal Medicine*, vol. 176, no. 1, January 2016, https://jamanetwork.com/journals/jamainternalmedicine/fullarticle/2467782.

[12] W. David Bradford, John Turner, and Jonathan W. Williams, "Off-Label Use of Pharmaceuticals: A Detection Controlled Estimation Approach," presentation at the Innovation and Behavior in Health Markets Conference, 2016, revised May 24, 2018, https://papers.ssrn.com/sol3/papers.cfm?abstract_id=2230976.

[13] Michael B. Shea, Mark Stewart, Hugo Van Dyke, Linda Ostermann, Jeff Allen, and Ellen Sigal, "Outdated Prescription Drug Labeling: How FDA-Approved Prescribing Information Lags Behind Real-World Clinical Practice," Therapeutic Innovation & Regulatory Science, vol. 52, issue 6 (first published online March 5, 2018; issue published November 1, 2018),

the 451 compendium-accepted uses, 56% were off-label. Of the off-label uses, the authors deemed 91% as "well-accepted off-label use."[14]

Labeling: History, Requirements, and Value

History

Drug labeling has been central to FDA's role as a protector of the public's health since 1906. That year, Congress (1) required that sellers state on a drug's label the "quantity or proportion of any alcohol [or] opium" contained, and (2) considered as "misbranded" any drug whose label was "false or misleading." Requirements that drugs be safe were not established until 1938. Congress did not require they be effective until 1962.[15]

Requirements

Today, a drug's labeling is more than the sticker the pharmacy places on the amber vial it dispenses to a customer.[16] The Federal Food, Drug, and Cosmetics Act (FFDCA) and associated FDA regulations[17] require and describe a product's labeling as "a compilation of information about the product, approved by FDA, based on the agency's thorough analysis of the new drug application (NDA) or biologics license application (BLA)

---

https://www.focr.org/sites/default/files/pdf/FOCR-Labeling-Research-Article.pdf?eType=EmailBlastContent&eId=067b86ca-de59-4767-86ab-8a4ad95a7978; abstract at https://journals.sagepub.com/doi/full/10.1177/2168479018759662.

14 The authors (Shea et al.) defined "well-accepted off-label drug use" if the National Comprehensive Cancer Network (NCCN) Drugs and Biologics Compendium graded the use in its top two categories of evidence.

15 Federal Food and Drug Act of 1906 (F&DA), P.L. 59-384, 1906; Federal Food, Drug, and Cosmetic Act (FFDCA), P.L. 75-717, 1938; and Kefauver-Harris Drug Amendments to the FFDCA, P.L. 87-781, 1962.

16 For examples of labeling, search for a drug at Drugs@FDA (https://www.accessdata.fda.gov/scripts/cder/daf/).

17 FFDCA Section 201(m), 21 C.F.R. Part 201—Labeling, and FDA, "[Docket No. 2000N–1269] (formerly Docket No. 00N–1269) RIN 0910–AA94, Requirements on Content and Format of Labeling for Human Prescription Drug and Biological Products," *Federal Register*, vol. 71, no. 15, January 24, 2006, pp. 3922-3997, http://www.gpo.gov/fdsys/pkg/FR-2006-01-24/pdf/06-545.pdf.

submitted by the applicant. This labeling contains information necessary for safe and effective use."

FDA requires that labeling begin with a highlights section that includes, if appropriate, black-box warnings, so called because their black borders signify importance.[18] The regulations list the required elements of labeling:[19]

• indications and usage • dosage and administration • dosage forms and strengths contraindications • warnings and precautions adverse reactions	• drug interactions • use in specific populations • drug abuse and dependence • overdosage • description • clinical pharmacology	• nonclinical toxicology • clinical studies • references • how supplied/storage and handling • patient counseling information

Value. Labeling plays a major role in the presentation of safety and effectiveness information. For clinicians, it is a primary source of prescribing information. The manufacturer submits the approved labeling for publication in the widely used *Physician's Desk Reference*. That labeling also serves as the basis for several patient-focused information sheets that manufacturers, pharmacy vendors, and many web-based drug information sites produce.[20]

---

[18] "Boxed warning. Certain contraindications or serious warnings, particularly those that may lead to death or serious injury, may be required by the FDA to be presented in a box" (21 C.F.R. 201.57(c)(1)).

[19] 21 C.F.R. 201.56(d). For older drugs, labeling content requirements are listed in 21 C.F.R. 201.56(e).

[20] PDR Network, http://www.pdr.net/about-pdr-network/. Examples of consumer medication information materials include those by Wolters Kluwer Health, Inc. (used, for example, with Target dispensing, http://www.consumerreports.org/health/best-buy-drugs/prescription-labels/patient-instructions/index.htm); First Databank, Inc. (provides FDA Medication Guides, http://www.fdbhealth.com/solutions/retail-pharmacy-dispensing/); and American Society of Health-System Pharmacists Consumer Medication Information (http://www.ahfsdruginformation.com/products_services/ahfs_cmi.aspx).

Off-Label Use: Description and Examples

Off-label prescribing can reflect cutting-edge clinical expertise. It can also be a response to price: a physician may choose to prescribe a lower-priced drug instead of a specifically labeled higher-priced one. Or a physician may prescribe off-label in an attempt to try a different treatment approach when other options have failed.

Sometimes an off-label use becomes so widespread that it becomes accepted practice. However, without the backing of carefully designed clinical trials and expert analysis, it remains unknown whether the drug is, in fact, safe and effective for the off-label use. Also unknown are dosing details and systematically evaluated associated adverse events.

Examples of off-label use include

- a drug tested for the treatment of one disease prescribed in an attempt to prevent or treat another;
- a drug tested at one dose used at higher or lower doses;
- a drug tested in adults prescribed to children; and
- a drug tested in an eight-week trial prescribed for long-term use.

Table 1 lists several examples of FDA-approved drugs widely prescribed for off-label uses.

Although FDA materials do not list off-label uses, several drug compendia include both labeled and off-label uses. For Medicare coverage, for example, the Social Security Act defines “medically accepted indication” as those, in addition to uses approved by FDA, that have been evaluated and supported and listed in one of several compendia, or for which there is “supportive clinical evidence in peer reviewed medical literature.”[21]

---

[21] Social Security Act §1861(t)(2)(B) [42 U.S.C. 1395x]. Compendia—available by subscription—include the American Hospital Formulary Service’s Drug Information, National Comprehensive Cancer Network Drug and Biologics Compendium, and Thomson Micromedex DrugDex.

Table 1. Selected Off-Label Uses

Drug	Labeled Uses	Off-Label Uses
gabapentin	post-herpetic pain; epilepsy seizures	peripheral diabetic neuropathy; menopausal hot flashes; attention deficit disorder; bipolar disorder
ketamine	anesthesia	depression, migraines
fentanyl	"management of pain in opioid-tolerant patients, severe enough to require daily, around-the-clock, long-term opioid treatment and for which alternative treatment options are inadequate"[a] "management of breakthrough pain in cancer patients … who are already receiving and who are tolerant to around-the-clock opioid therapy for their underlying persistent cancer pain"[b]	less severe or chronic pain; for individuals who are not opioid-tolerant
antipsychotics (e.g., risperidone, olanzapine, quetiapine)	schizophrenia; bipolar disorder	sleep aid; behavioral symptoms of dementia; obsessive compulsive disorder, posttraumatic stress syndrome, anxiety disorders[c]
methylphenidate	attention deficit disorders in children; narcolepsy[d]	attention deficit disorders in adults, depression, autism spectrum disorder
Avastin	certain non-squamous non-small cell lung cancer; glioblastoma, renal cell carcinoma, cervical cancer, epithelial ovarian, fallopian tube, or primary peritoneal cancer	wet age-related macular degeneration; colorectal cancer

Source: Labeled uses excerpted from FDA-approved labeling posted at Drugs@FDA (https://www.accessdata.fda.gov/scripts/cder/daf/). Examples of off-label uses compiled by CRS based on clinical databases and news accounts.

[a] Labeling for Duragesic (transdermal), a brand-name fentanyl product.

[b] Labeling for Subsys (sublingual), a brand-name fentanyl product.

[c] "Off-Label Use of Atypical Antipsychotics: An Update," Comparative Effectiveness Review No. 43, John M.

Eisenberg Center for Clinical Decisions and Communications Science, August 1, 2012, http://www.effectivehealthcare.ahrq.gov/offlabelantipsych.cfm.

[d] Labeling from Ritalin, a brand-name methylphenidate product.

BENEFITS AND RISKS OF OFF-LABEL USE

Why has Congress given FDA the authority to regulate whether a drug may be on the U.S. market? Two key reasons: to protect patients and to encourage research in a competitive pharmaceutical industry.[22]

By statute and regulation, FDA now approves a drug for a specific use once its sponsor (usually the manufacturer) has provided sufficient evidence that the drug is safe and effective for that use. FDA has developed procedures for the review of that evidence. The FDA-approved labeling, which informs the clinician about dosing and likely and unlikely adverse events, helps protect the individuals for whom the drug is prescribed.

Labeling also helps protect the interests of the manufacturers who invest in the clinical trials that demonstrate safety and effectiveness. For new drugs and new uses of already approved drugs, the sponsor receives a period of market protection, in the form of regulatory exclusivity for the sale of the drug for those uses. Payors—such as private health insurers or Medicare—benefit from FDA-approved labeling in their evaluation of whether to pay for a drug's use.

But use of a drug evolves as clinicians (and the manufacturer) share their experiences regarding off-label uses, which, by definition, were not part of the premarket clinical studies used to obtain FDA approval. Off-label use can benefit patients. In some instances, such as in the treatment of rare diseases, clinical practice may use drugs approved for other indications. A manufacturer may choose not to invest in trials for such a small patient group.[23] A patient whose physician is already prescribing the drug off-label may not want to enroll in a clinical trial where there is a chance he or she may be assigned to the placebo group. Once drugs are well-established in off-label uses, manufacturers rarely design studies to determine or verify the

---

[22] FDA statement at https://www.fda.gov/AboutFDA/Transparency/Basics/ucm194877.htm; and FFDCA §1003 [21 U.S.C. 393].

[23] See, for example, testimony to FDA by the National Organization for Rare Disorders, November 9, 2016, https://rarediseases.org/wp-content/uploads/2014/11/2016-11-09.-NORD-Statement-at-FDA-Off-Label-PublicHearing.pdf.

safety and effectiveness of such uses. Individuals and groups wanting to conduct such studies may find it hard to obtain funding.

Examples of adverse events (AEs) associated with the use of drugs for specific off-label uses include heart valve damage from the use of fenfluramine and phentermine (fen-phen) for weight loss, and seizures from the use of tiagabine hydrochloride for depression.[24] Using a Canadian primary care database that captured all prescriptions, the reason for each prescription, and adverse events, researchers looked at the rate of AEs for on-label use, off-label use associated with "strong scientific evidence," and off-label use without such evidence. They found more AEs for off-label prescriptions than for on-label prescriptions. However, off-label use associated with strong scientific evidence had similar rates of AEs as did on-label uses. The increased risk of AEs for off-label use was concentrated in those uses without strong scientific evidence.[25]

Manufacturers benefit from sales for off-label uses. However, they risk losing that market should a competitor complete studies to obtain FDA approval and labeling for those uses. Researchers who are not supported by the manufacturer who try to assess the safety and effectiveness of off-label uses are hampered by the inexact nature of secondary data sources: the standard clinical trial data collection in preparation for an FDA application is not available for off-label uses. What may begin as hopeful and intermittent off-label use may gain momentum and offer opportunities for planned studies.

Drug and device companies argue that current regulations prevent them from distributing important information to physicians and payors about unapproved, off-label uses of their products.[26] In November 2016, FDA held a two-day public meeting to hear from various groups regarding

---

[24] Tewodros Eguale, David L. Buckeridge, Aman Verma, Nancy E. Winslade, Andrea Benedetti, James A. Hanley, Robyn Tamblyn, "Association of Off-label Drug Use and Adverse Drug Events in an Adult Population," *JAMA Internal Medicine*, vol. 176, no. 1, January 2016, https://jamanetwork.com/journals/jamainternalmedicine/fullarticle/2467782.

[25] Tewodros Eguale, David L. Buckeridge, Aman Verma, Nancy E. Winslade, Andrea Benedetti, James A. Hanley, Robyn Tamblyn, "Association of Off-label Drug Use and Adverse Drug Events in an Adult Population," *JAMA Internal Medicine*, vol. 176, no. 1, January 2016, https://jamanetwork.com/journals/jamainternalmedicine/fullarticle/ 2467782.

[26] STAT, "FDA to hold long-awaited meeting to review off-label marketing," August 31, 2016, https://www.statnews.com/pharmalot/2016/05/27/fda-hhs-free-speech-patient-safety/.

off-label uses of approved or cleared medical products.[27] In June 2018, FDA issued final guidances explaining the agency's policy about medical product communications that include data and information not contained in FDA-approved labeling.[28]

One FDA guidance document, in particular, described the types of information that a manufacturer could provide payors and formulary committees about unapproved uses of approved products.[29] FDA made two points especially relevant to off-label uses.

First, FDA differentiates among its audiences in its presentation of information. The material it allows in product labeling is directed to a clinical audience. FDA staff have reviewed the information and require that it be presented in a way that is understandable by individual clinicians, who often do not have the statistical sophistication or data analysis skills or resources to fully evaluate the claims of manufacturers. This guidance notes, though, that payors and formulary committees do have such expertise and resources. FDA also acknowledges that it is useful for payors to have information in their decisions on coverage, but it wants to ensure that the information manufacturers provide is not misleading.

Second, the FDA guidance describes what harm could come from allowing more sharing of information about off-label use.

---

[27] FDA, Docket No. FDA-2016-N-1149, https://s3.amazonaws.com/public-inspection.federal register.gov/2016- 21062.pdf. All prescription drugs must receive FDA approval for marketing. About 1% of medical devices go through a comparable approval process; most devices receive FDA clearance for marketing. For a description of FDA medical device regulation, see CRS Report R42130, *FDA Regulation of Medical Devices*.

[28] FDA, "Guidance for Industry: Medical Product Communications That Are Consistent With the FDA-Required Labeling—Questions and Answers," Center for Drug Evaluation and Research, Center for Biologics Evaluation and Research, Center for Devices and Radiological Health, Center for Veterinary Medicine, and Office of the Commissioner, June 2018, https://www.fda.gov/downloads/drugs/guidancecomplianceregulatoryinformation/ guidances/ucm537130.pdf.

[29] FDA, "Guidance for Industry and Review Staff: Drug and Device Manufacturer Communications With Payors, Formulary Committees, and Similar Entities—Questions and Answers," Center for Drug Evaluation and Research, Center for Biologics Evaluation and Research, Center for Devices and Radiological Health, and Office of the Commissioner, June 2018, https://www.fda.gov/downloads/Drugs/GuidanceComplianceRegulatoryInformation/ Guidances/UCM537347.pdf.

> Some firm communications regarding unapproved products or unapproved uses of approved/cleared/licensed medical products may potentially undermine substantial government interests related to health and safety. These interests include motivating the development of robust scientific data on safety and efficacy; maintaining the premarket review process for safety and efficacy of each intended use in order to prevent harm, to protect against fraud, misrepresentation, and bias, and to develop appropriate instructions for use for medical products; protecting the integrity and reliability of promotional information regarding medical product uses; and preventing the diversion of health care resources toward ineffective treatments.

The concerns FDA raised in the June 2018 final guidance documents might explain why Congress may be interested in exploring the issue of off-label use further.

History of Congressional Interest and Action

Congress has developed a system to protect the public by ensuring that drugs sold in the United States have met clinical and manufacturing standards of safety and effectiveness. Labeling is the mechanism that bridges the regulated drug and the use of that drug in clinical practice. The labeling establishes the uses for which the manufacturer has demonstrated safety and effectiveness to FDA's satisfaction. Congress and the FDA have tried several approaches, using labeling as a tool, to reduce the risk to patients. *Table A-1* includes examples of congressional and FDA actions to expand the information provided in a drug's labeling. The actions have addressed topics such as

- content labeling,
- directions for use,
- permissible and prohibited advertising,
- research incentives to support labeling specific to population subgroups (e.g., children),

- criteria for Medicare coverage,
- required and permissible labeling changes, and
- balance of benefit and risk information in labeling and advertising.

Manufacturers, meanwhile, want to be able to provide information to insurers and other entities (such as the Centers for Medicare and Medicaid Services [CMS] and hospital pharmacy and therapeutics committees) that decide whether to cover a drug in a policy and whether to limit reimbursement for specific uses. Congress has provided some leeway relative to its earlier prohibition on promotional activities. For example, in 2016, it broadened the types of health care economic information drug and device manufacturers could provide to payors (e.g., insurance companies).[30] Although the underlying FFDCA section continues to exclude information related only to an off-label use, it now requires "a conspicuous and prominent statement describing any material differences between the health care economic information and the labeling approved for the drug." Several bills concerning off-label use have been introduced that would have expanded the information that manufacturers could provide about off-label uses. For example, the Subcommittee on Health of the House Committee on Energy and Commerce marked up H.R. 2026 (115th Congress), the Pharmaceutical Information Exchange Act, in January 2018, which would have allowed the provision of *scientific information* to payors, in addition to health care economic information.[31] Then-Subcommittee Chair Michael Burgess, in commenting on the bill's effort to clarify how manufacturers can share "if it is based on competent and reliable evidence," expressed strong support for the bill. He noted "the importance of cutting edge information in medicine and science to

---

[30] Sec. 3037 of P.L. 114-255, the 21st Century Cures Act.

[31] Subcommittee on Health, House Committee on Energy and Commerce, mark-up of H.R. 2026, January 17, 2018, https://energycommerce.house.gov/committee-activity/markups/markup-of-hr-over-the-counter-monograph-safetyinnovation-and-reform-act.

optimize patient care and outcomes ... and [how the bill] could have the potential to save patients' lives."[32]

Then-Ranking Member (now, Chair) Frank Pallone, Jr., though, argued that the ability to communicate about off-label use "had great potential to undermine" FDA's approval process and to "hamstring" its enforcement efforts.[33] H.R. 2026 passed the subcommittee, although it did not reach the floor in the 115th Congress.

POSSIBLE AVENUES OF FUTURE CONGRESSIONAL INTEREST

Off-label use presents both opportunities and risks to clinicians, patients, manufacturers, and researchers. At times, those interests clash. Academics, public health organizations, and journals have suggested what actions Congress might take based on their particular concerns regarding off-label prescriptions.[34] These actions include both direct legislation and oversight activities to encourage action by other entities. The 116th Congress might consider some of these varied approaches, summarized in the issues described below.

---

[32] Subcommittee on Health, House Committee on Energy and Commerce, mark-up of H.R. 2026, January 17, 2018, https://energycommerce.house.gov/committee-activity/markups/markup-of-hr-over-the-counter-monograph-safetyinnovation-and-reform-act.

[33] Subcommittee on Health, House Committee on Energy and Commerce, mark-up of H.R. 2026, January 17, 2018, https://energycommerce.house.gov/committee-activity/markups/markup-of-hr-over-the-counter-monograph-safetyinnovation-and-reform-act.

[34] For example: Zachary Brennan, "New Report Investigates Drivers of Off-Label Prescribing in the EU," Regulatory Focus, March 3, 2017; Christine Fukada, Jillian Clare Kohler, Heather Boon, Zubin Austin, and Murray Krahn, "Prescribing gabapentin off label: Perspectives from psychiatry, pain and neurology specialists," CPJ/RPC, vol. 145, no. 6, November/December 2012; Megan Thielking, "A STAT Investigation: Ketamine gives hope to patients with severe depression. But some clinics stray from the science and hype its benefits," STAT, September 24, 2018, https://www.statnews.com/2018/09/24/ketamine-clinics-severe-depression-treatment; and Joshua D. Wallach and Joseph S. Ross, "Gabapentin Approvals, Off-Label Use, and Lessons from Postmarketing Evaluation Efforts," *JAMA*, vol. 319, no. 8, February 27, 2018.

Disclosure to Patients

Most individuals, unaware of the nuances of FDA regulation, may not know that physicians may prescribe drugs for uses that FDA has not reviewed for safety and effectiveness. Several potential opportunities for providing this information exist. Congress could require or work with the states to require that

- the prescriber inform the patient about the off-label use and describe the meaning of off-label use;
- the prescriber note in the prescription why the drug is being prescribed; or
- the pharmacist inform the patient that the use is off-label.

Data Collection and Availability

FDA, under federal law, determines whether a drug requires a prescription. The states, under their individual laws, determine what information the prescription order contains. Because clinicians do not need to note on the prescription order why they are prescribing a drug (e.g., simvastatin for high cholesterol or citalopram for depression), the information in pharmacy, administrative, and clinical databases often cannot directly identify off-label uses. Therefore, as Congress and other public policy groups consider whether and how to address off-label drug prescribing, they do not have adequate information on the scope and details of the practice. Congress could require or work with the states to encourage

- clinicians to note on prescriptions the reason for medication use (e.g., the specific condition, disease, or symptom), thereby allowing that information to appear in pharmacy databases, which would enable focused analysis of off-label uses;

- the establishment of confidential registries of off-label prescribing and follow-up information that FDA (or other designated scientifically appropriate agencies) could use in its electronic surveillance systems to identify associated adverse events and other drug use problems; or
- FDA to increase its surveillance of available data sources, such as registries and administrative and clinical databases, to identify patterns of off-label use and evidence suggesting effectiveness and associated adverse events.

Dissemination

Because some information may be valuable to clinicians and entities that influence prescribing decisions (such as insurers and pharmacy and therapeutics committees), Congress could allow manufacturers to disseminate information about off-label uses that they have developed or of which they are aware, perhaps subject to certain limitations or accompanying reporting requirements. Possibilities include broader sharing of clinical analyses of off-label use with coverage deciders (e.g., CMS, insurers, pharmacy and therapeutics committees) to support requests that they cover a particular use of the drug; and dissemination of clinical analyses of off-label use at clinical and pharmaceutical conferences.

Oversight

With an estimated 12% to 38% of all prescriptions' (and 56% of oncology prescriptions') being written for uses not listed on FDA-approved labeling,[35] valid information on the extent of off-label use and

---

[35] David C. Radley, Stan N. Finkelstein, and Randall S. Stafford, "Off-label Prescribing Among Office-Based Physicians," Archives of Internal Medicine, vol. 166, May 8, 2006; Tewodros Eguale, David L. Buckeridge, Aman Verma, Nancy E. Winslade, Andrea Benedetti, James A. Hanley, Robyn Tamblyn, "Association of Off-label Drug Use and Adverse Drug Events

the effect of such use on manufacturer, insurer, and clinician behavior could potentially better inform debate on how to best protect the public's health. Congress could direct

- the Government Accountability Office (GAO) to study the extent of off-label use in government-provided care (e.g., Department of Veterans Affairs, Bureau of Prisons, and Indian Health Service) and in government-funded care (e.g., Medicare and Medicaid);
- the Secretary of Health and Human Services (HHS) to contract with the National Academy of Medicine or a similar organization to assemble management or industrial policy experts to study the costs and rewards to industry of off-label prescriptions; or
- FDA and the Federal Trade Commission to investigate drugs whose off-label prescriptions account for a particularly high percentage of all prescriptions or that generate a particularly high percentage or high dollar value of sales.

Pricing

The decision to use a drug off-label based solely or primarily on price introduces a new element to study. For example, the pricing difference between Avastin and Lucentis, both made by the same manufacturer with the same active ingredient, is so large that many ophthalmologists use the

---

in an Adult Population," *JAMA Internal Medicine*, vol. 176, no. 1, January 2016, https://jamanetwork.com/journals/jamainternalmedicine/fullarticle/2467782; W. David Bradford, John Turner, and Jonathan W. Williams, "Off-Label Use of Pharmaceuticals: A Detection Controlled Estimation Approach," presentation at the Innovation and Behavior in Health Markets Conference, 2016, revised May 24, 2018, https://papers.ssrn.com/sol3/papers.cfm?abstract_id=2230976; Michael B. Shea, Mark Stewart, Hugo Van Dyke, Linda Ostermann, Jeff Allen, and Ellen Sigal, "Outdated Prescription Drug Labeling: How FDA-Approved Prescribing Information Lags Behind Real-World Clinical Practice," Therapeutic Innovation & Regulatory Science, vol. 52, issue 6 (first published online March 5, 2018; issue published November 1, 2018), https://www.focr.org/sites/default/files/pdf/FOCR-Labeling-Research-Article.pdf?eType=EmailBlastContent&eId=067b86ca-de59-4767-86ab-8a4ad95a7978; abstract at https://journals.sagepub.com/doi/full/10.1177/2168479018759662.

lower priced Avastin in their treatment of macular degeneration, despite its being an off-label use.[36] The manufacturer included the treatment of macular degeneration in its application to FDA for Lucentis. To explore the ramifications of a traditionally nonclinical element in prescribing decisions, Congress could require

- the HHS Secretary to study the relationship among pricing, access, and prescribing and its effect on patient safety.

Reimbursement

Although FDA approval of a drug—not for each use of a drug—is a requirement for sale in the United States, the decision to reimburse a physician or patient for a drug is made by entities such as the CMS and private insurers. Such decisions, therefore, influence what drugs are prescribed and, in part, for what uses drugs are prescribed. Congress could direct

- the HHS Secretary to study such coverage decisions or to contract with the National Academy of Medicine or a similarly equipped entity to do so; or
- HHS to form a task force to include CMS and FDA, along with private insurers and others involved in coverage decisions, and patient and clinician groups representing those affected by coverage decisions, to identify areas in need of action and to recommend steps in those directions.

Congress also could encourage

- payors to require safety and effectiveness evidence before covering off-label uses.

---

[36] Kierstan Boyd, "What Is Avastin?" American Academy of Ophthalmology, May 17, 2018, https://www.aao.org/eyehealth/diseases/amd-macular-degeneration.

Research

The traditional path toward adding an indication (reason for use) to the labeling of a drug already approved for other uses has been for the sponsor of the drug to conduct clinical trials and submit a supplemental new drug application (NDA) to FDA. The widespread extent of off-label use suggests that relying on that model is not helping prescribers get better information. Congress could consider

- assigning responsibility (and funding) to the National Institutes of Health and the Patient-Centered Outcomes Research Institute for safety and effectiveness evaluations of off-label uses; or
- requiring, for a drug that has substantial (to be defined) off-label sales, that the manufacturer[37] fund studies, such as clinical trials, to assess the safety and effectiveness of the drug for the off-label use and submit evidence to the HHS Secretary. Depending on the Secretary's assessment of the evidence, the Secretary could request that the manufacturer amend the drug's labeling either to add the off-label use to the label as an approved use or to add a statement that clinical evidence does not support the safety and effectiveness of the drug for the off-label use.

Research Transparency

FDA regulations describe standards for the design and analysis of clinical trials that a sponsor uses in an NDA. Studies done by or for the manufacturer or by other groups or individuals are not always made public, in which case their findings cannot be reviewed and evaluated.

---

[37] For drugs on patent, this would be the brand-name sponsor of the new drug application (NDA). For drugs no longer on patent that are only marketed as generic products, this would be the holder of the abbreviated NDA. For a description of the regulation of generic drugs, see CRS Report R44703, *Generic Drugs and GDUFA Reauthorization: In Brief.*

Because the results of such studies may be used in support of off-label uses, by providing positive and negative incentives, Congress could consider requiring or encouraging

- prospective posting of the designs and statistical plans of studies of off-label uses; or
- public reporting of studies of off-label use.

Clinical Guidance

Professional societies and other clinical groups often supplement the information available to prescribers from FDA-approved labeling, medical journals, and information from manufacturers. They can issue guidelines and recommend best practices. Congress could engage such groups and encourage

- professional societies to develop evidence-based clinical guidelines and training regarding off-label use.

Precedents from Other Countries

The United States is not alone in facing the health care and economic implications of off-label use. For example, the member countries of the European Union have addressed measures involving reimbursement, guidance for prescribers, professional standards, and informed consent.[38] Congress could require

[38] Zachary Brennan, "New Report Investigates Drivers of Off-Label Prescribing in the EU," Regulatory Focus, March 3, 2017.

- HHS to contract with the National Academy of Medicine or a similarly equipped entity to review measures taken by the European Union and other regulatory bodies and recommend legislative or administrative actions as appropriate.

CONCLUDING COMMENTS

Concerns over off-label use overlap with questions raised by some legislators and regulators in other contexts. In addition to clearly related issues such as what is allowable information in direct-to-consumer advertising, promotion to clinicians, and material shared with payors and insurers, off-label use also affects the entire basis of FDA regulation of drugs through its authority to approve drugs. That means it directly or indirectly affects research, clinical innovation, transparency, patents and exclusivities, pricing, and access.

Changes in law or regulation in any one area may have benefits in some areas and drawbacks in others. For example, FDA's initiative to encourage research in drugs used traditionally but never reviewed and approved by FDA—so-called legacy drugs—stems from its desire for evidence of safety and effectiveness.[39] Such evidence helps protect patients from possible use of ineffective, unsafe, or misdosed drugs. That initiative, in turn, helps enable sponsors to conduct the clinical trials, submit new drug applications, obtain regulatory exclusivity with the new drug approval— and then raise the price of the new branded product while expecting FDA to honor the exclusivity and block the sale of the drug by others. For example, clinicians had been prescribing a compounded version of progestin for use in preventing preterm delivery. Such use had never been adequately tested in clinical trials. One company conducted those

---

[39] FDA, Unapproved Drugs Initiative, https://www.fda.gov/Drugs/GuidanceCompliance RegulatoryInformation/EnforcementActivitiesbyFDA/SelectedEnforcementActionsonUnap provedDrugs/ucm118990.htm Guidance for FDA Staff and Industry, and FDA "Marketed Unapproved Drugs—Compliance Policy Guide Sec. 440.100 Marketed New Drugs without Approved NDAs or ANDAs," September 19, 2011, https://www.fda.gov/downloads/drugs/ guidance complianceregulatoryinformation/guidances/ucm070290.pdf.

trials, and FDA approved its new drug application. The initial price for the new drug, Makena, was $30,000 for a 20-week course; patients had been paying pharmacists $200-$400 for the same course.[40] Unanticipated price increases can also arise from the apparent following of FDA procedures. For example, a new owner of the FDA-approval of an old antiparasitic generic drug raised the price from $14 per tablet to $750, Daraprim's initial price.[41] Such sudden and large price increases become a barrier to patient access and, therefore, a potential threat to health.

In the case of off-label prescribing, actions in any direction—whether by Congress, FDA, or the courts—could have both intended and unanticipated effects. Actions to limit off-label prescribing could have the intended effects of reducing safety risks and the economic cost of using drugs ineffective for their prescribed purposes. Such limits, however, could also stifle informed clinical exploration. Similarly, incentives to mount clinical trials needed to add an indication to the label could help identify and disseminate information on dosing and contradictions. Such incentives, however, could also hurt. For example, a brand drug that added a new indication to its labeling could prevent, through exclusivities, generics from similarly modifying their labeling. Patients could need to pay more.

---

[40] Joanne Armstrong, "Unintended Consequences—The Cost of Preventing Preterm Births after FDA Approval of a Branded Version of 17OHP," *New England Journal of Medicine,* online March 16, 2011; and Gardiner Harris, "Drugs' Cost and Safety Fuel a Fight," *New York Times*, April 4, 2011, https://www.nytimes.com/2011/04/05/health/05FDA.html?rref=collection%2Fbyline%2Fgardiner-harris&action=click&contentCollection=undefined &region=stream&module=stream_unit&version=search&contentPlacement=1&pgtype=coll ection. The compounded version of the drug continues to be available for indications other than prevention of prematurity. FDA has not actively sought to stop sales. See Yesha Patel and Martha M. Rumore, Controversies in Practice "Hydroxyprogesterone Caproate Injection (Makena) One Year Later: To Compound or Not to Compound—That Is the Question," P&T, vol. 37 no. 7, July 2012, pp. 405-411, https://www.ncbi. nlm.nih.gov/ pmc/articles/PMC3411212/pdf/ptj3707405.pdf, and FDA, "Questions and Answers on Updated FDA Statement on Compounded Versions of hydroxyprogesterone caproate (the active ingredient in Makena)," Press Announcement, Page Last Updated: 06/29/2012, http://wayback.archive-it.org/7993/20170113105722/http://www.fda.gov/NewsEvents/ Newsroom/PressAnnouncements/ucm310215.htm.

[41] Andrew Pollack, "Drug Goes From $13.50 a Tablet to $750, Overnight," *New York Times*, September 20, 2015, https://www.nytimes.com/2015/09/21/business/a-huge-overnight-increase-in-a-drugs-price-raises-protests.html.

The recent debates over the right-to-try movement regarding use of investigational drugs by terminally ill patients[42] may preview discussion about any proposed restrictions on off-label use. The Goldwater Institute, considered a key impetus to development and passage of the 2018 enactment of a right-to-try act,[43] looks to diminish government's role in an individual's choice and has supported dissemination of off-label information.[44]

Congress has built a process in which a robust FDA can regulate drugs to protect the public's health. Is there cause for concern that perhaps a third[45] of prescriptions are for off-label uses and that, in at least one study, three-quarters of those had minimal or no accepted scientific evidence to support their use?[46]

Policy tension exists over the line between wanting to ensure individuals' freedom to take drugs for off-label uses and wanting to protect the public from the risk of unsafe or ineffective drugs. Where to draw that line—and how to know when it may be time to move the line—is of continuing interest to regulators and legislators.

---

[42] CRS Report R45414, Right to Try: Access to Investigational Drugs.

[43] See, for example, ADI News Services, "Goldwater Institute's Right To Try Bill Signed By California Governor," Arizona Daily Independent, September 29, 2016, https://arizonadailyindependent.com/2016/09/29/goldwater-institutesright-to-try-bill-signed-by-california-governor/; and Marie McCullough, "For the terminally ill, are 'right-to-try' laws offering a lifeline, or false hope?" The [Philadelphia] Inquirer, April 4, 2017, https://www.philly.com/philly/health/Do-Right-to-Try-laws-offer-a-lifeline-or-false-hope-to-the-terminally-ill.html.

[44] Naomi Lopez Bauman, "Restoring Free Speech in Medicine," Goldwater Institute, June 6, 2017, https://goldwaterinstitute.org/article/restoring-free-speech-in-medicine; and Starlee Coleman, "Arizona becomes first state to allow pharmaceutical companies to legally communicate off-label treatment uses to medical professionals," Goldwater Institute, March 23, 2017, https://goldwaterinstitute.org/article/arizona-becomes-first-state-to-allow-pharmaceutical-companies-legally-communicate-off-label-treatment/.

[45] W. David Bradford, John Turner, and Jonathan W. Williams, "Off-Label Use of Pharmaceuticals: A Detection Controlled Estimation Approach," presentation at the Innovation and Behavior in Health Markets Conference, 2016, revised May 24, 2018, https://papers.ssrn.com/sol3/papers.cfm?abstract_id=2230976.

[46] David C. Radley, Stan N. Finkelstein, and Randall S. Stafford, "Off-label Prescribing Among Office-Based Physicians," Archives of Internal Medicine, vol. 166, May 8, 2006.

APPENDIX. SELECTED ACTIONS TO EXPAND INFORMATION IN DRUG LABELING

Table A-1. Selected Congressional and FDA Actions to Expand Information in Drug Labeling

Date	Topic	Law or Agency Action
1906	Required that sellers state on a drug's label the "quantity or proportion of any alcohol, opium, ..." contained; and considered as "misbranded" any drug whose label was "false or misleading."	Federal Food and Drug Act of 1906 (F&DA), P.L. 59-384
1938	Required that labeling include adequate directions for use and evidence of safety of their labeled use.	Federal Food, Drug, and Cosmetic Act (FFDCA), P.L. 75-717
1962	Would declare as misbranded a prescription drug whose advertising did not adhere to required labeling information.	Kefauver-Harris Drug Amendments to the FFDCA, P.L. 87-781. Sec. 131 added FFDCA Sec. 502(n).
1975	Prohibited manufacturers from advertising and otherwise promoting off-label uses of approved drugs.	21 CFR 202.1, Prescription drug advertisements [40 FR 14016, March 27, 1975]
1977–2003	FDA issued a 1977 guidance and a 1998 rule, and Congress took up related efforts in 2002 and 2003 to both require and encourage manufacturers to conduct the research to support adequate labeling concerning the use for children of approved drugs.	FDA, "Guidance for Industry: General Considerations for the Clinical Evaluation of Drugs in Infants and Children," September 1977, http://www.fda.gov/downloads/Drugs/GuidanceComplianceRegulatoryInformation/ Guidances/ucm071687.pdf; FDA, "Regulations Requiring Manufacturers to Assess the Safety and Effectiveness of New Drugs and Biological Products in Pediatric Patients; Final rule," Federal Register, vol. 63, no. 231, December 2, 1998, pp. 66632-66672; Best Pharmaceuticals for Children Act (BPCA, P.L. 107-109); and Pediatric Research Equity Act (PREA, P.L. 108-155).
1993	Added Medicare coverage of off-label cancer drug use, by defining "medically accepted indication" as, for an FDA-approved drug, a use included in a cited compendia or other Secretary-defined compendia or which the carrier determines is acceptable based peer-reviewed supportive clinical evidence according to guidance from the Secretary.	P.L. 103-66 amended the Social Security Act Sec. 1861(t)(2)(B) [42 U.S.C. 1395x].

Date	Topic	Law or Agency Action
1993–2007	FDA issued "Guideline for the Study and Evaluation of Gender Differences in the Clinical Evaluation of Drugs." Directed the Secretary of Health and Human Services to review and develop guidance on including women and minorities in clinical trials, which would make appropriate labeling possible.	FDA, "Guideline for the Study and Evaluation of Gender Differences in the Clinical Evaluation of Drugs," Federal Register, Vol. 58, No. 139, July 22, 1993. FDA Modernization Act of 1997 IFDAMA), P.L. 105-115
2006	Required that labeling include highlights of prescribing information to help health care providers use the information.	"Requirements on Content and Format of Labeling for Human Prescription Drug and Biological Products," referred to as the "Physician Labeling Rule," 71 FR 3922, January 24, 2006, 21 CFR 201.56 and 201.57.
2007	Authorized the Secretary, upon learning of new relevant safety information, to require a labeling change.	FDA Amendments Act of 2007, P.L. 110-85. See FFDCA 505(o).
2012	Directed the Secretary of Health and Human Services to assess the extent to which demographic subgroups (to include sex, age, race, and ethnicity) participate in clinical trials and are included in safety and effectiveness data submitted in marketing applications. It also required the Secretary to publish an action plan with recommendations to improve the completeness, quality, and inclusion of subgroup data in various analyses. Such information could then be reflected in a drug's labeling.	FDA Safety and Innovation Act (FDASIA), P.L. 112-144
2014	Required that labeling include a summary of the risks of using a drug during pregnancy and lactation	"Content and Format of Labeling for Human Prescription Drug and Biological Products; Requirements for Pregnancy and Lactation Labeling," referred to as the "Pregnancy and Lactation Labeling Rule," 79 FR 72063, December 4, 2014.
2016	Required FDA to establish a program to evaluate the use of real world evidence (RWE) to support approval of a new indication for an already approved drug.	Section 3022 of the 21st Century Cures Act, P.L. 114-255

Source: Compiled by CRS.

In: Key Congressional Reports for June 2019 ISBN: 978-1-53616-665-1
Editor: Amada A. Byrd

Chapter 2

MEDICAID: AN OVERVIEW (UPDATED)*

Alison Mitchell, Evelyne P. Baumrucker, Kirsten J. Colello, Angela Napili, Cliff Binder and Kirsten J. Colello

SUMMARY

Medicaid is a means-tested entitlement program that finances the delivery of primary and acute medical services as well as long-term services and supports (LTSS) to an estimated 75 million people at a cost to states and the federal government of $616 billion in FY2018. Medicaid is one of the largest payers in the U.S. health care system, representing 17% of national health care spending in CY2017; in that year, private health insurance and Medicare accounted for 34% and 20% of national health care spending, respectively.

Participation in Medicaid is voluntary for states, though all states, the District of Columbia, and the territories choose to participate. The federal government requires states to cover certain mandatory populations and services, but the federal government also allows states to cover other optional populations and services.

---

* This is an edited, reformatted and augmented version of Congressional Research Service Publication No. R43357, Updated June 24, 2019.

Due to this flexibility, there is substantial variation among the states in terms of factors such as Medicaid eligibility, covered benefits, and provider payment rates.

Historically, Medicaid eligibility generally has been limited to low-income children, pregnant women, parents of dependent children, the elderly, and individuals with disabilities; however, since 2014, states have had the option to cover nonelderly adults with income up to 133% of the federal poverty level (FPL) under the Patient Protection and Affordable Care Act (ACA; P.L. 111- 148, as amended) Medicaid expansion.

Medicaid coverage includes a variety of primary and acute-care services as well as LTSS. Not all Medicaid enrollees have access to the same set of services. An enrollee's eligibility pathway determines the available services within a benefit package. Federal law provides two primary benefit packages for state Medicaid programs: (1) traditional benefits and (2) alternative benefit plans (ABPs). Beneficiary cost sharing (e.g., premiums and co-payments) is limited under the Medicaid program.

Medicaid enrollees generally receive benefits via one of two service delivery systems: fee-forservice (FFS) or managed care. Under FFS, health care providers are paid by the state Medicaid program for each service provided to a Medicaid enrollee. Under managed care, Medicaid enrollees get most or all of their services through an organization under contract with the state. Most states use a combination of FFS and managed care.

The federal government and the states jointly finance Medicaid. The federal government reimburses states for a portion of each state's Medicaid program costs. Federal Medicaid funding is an open-ended entitlement to states, which means there is no upper limit or cap on the amount of federal Medicaid funds a state may receive.

The Social Security Act authorizes several waiver and demonstration authorities that allow states to operate their Medicaid programs outside of federal rules. The primary Medicaid waiver authorities include Section 1115, Section 1915(b), and Section 1915(c).

Medicaid provider payment rates are set by states within federal rules. In some cases, states make supplemental payments to Medicaid providers that are separate from, and in addition to, the payment rates for services rendered to Medicaid enrollees. Also, Medicaid program integrity initiatives are designed to combat fraud, waste, and abuse in the Medicaid program.

INTRODUCTION

Medicaid is a joint federal-state program that finances the delivery of primary and acute medical services, as well as long-term services and supports (LTSS), to a diverse low-income population, including children, pregnant women, adults, individuals with disabilities, and people aged 65 and older.

State participation in Medicaid is voluntary, although all states, the District of Columbia, and the territories[1] choose to participate. States must follow broad federal rules to receive federal matching funds, but they have flexibility to design their own versions of Medicaid within the federal statute's basic framework. This flexibility results in variability across state Medicaid programs.

The federal government and the states jointly finance the Medicaid program. Federal Medicaid spending is an entitlement, with total expenditures dependent on state policy decisions and use of services by enrollees. Medicaid is an entitlement for both states and individuals. The Medicaid entitlement to states ensures that, so long as states operate their programs within the federal requirements, states are entitled to federal Medicaid matching funds. Medicaid also is an individual entitlement, which means that anyone eligible and enrolled in Medicaid under his or her state's eligibility standards is guaranteed Medicaid coverage.

In FY2018, Medicaid is estimated to have provided health care services to almost 75 million individuals at a total cost of $616 billion, with the federal government paying $386 billion of that total.[2] In comparison, the Medicare program provided health care benefits to nearly 59 million individuals in that same year at a cost of roughly $711 billion.[3]

---

[1] The five territories are American Samoa, Guam, the Commonwealth of the Northern Mariana Islands, Puerto Rico, and the U.S. Virgin Islands..

[2] This enrollment figure is from Christopher J. Truffer, Christian J. Wolfe, and Kathryn E. Rennie, *2017 Actuarial Report on the Financial Outlook for Medicaid*, Office of the Actuary, Centers for Medicare & Medicaid Services (CMS), U.S. Department of Health & Human Services (HHS), 2018. The expenditures figures are from CMS, CMS-64 data as of April 29, 2019.

[3] Congressional Budget Office, "Medicare – CBO's May 2019 Baseline," May 2, 2019.

Medicaid provides a health care safety net for low-income populations,[4] with approximately 21% of the U.S. population with Medicaid coverage in 2017.[5] Medicaid plays a more significant role for certain subpopulations. For example, in 2017, Medicaid provided health coverage for 39% of all children in the United States;[6] in the same year, it provided health coverage for 61% of all nonelderly individuals with income below 100% of the federal poverty level (FPL).[7]

For some types of services, Medicaid is a significant payer. For instance, in 2017, Medicaid accounted for about 44% of national spending on LTSS.[8] Medicaid paid for 43% of all births in the United States in 2017.[9] In FY2015, Medicaid accounted for 75% of public family planning expenditures (including federal, state, and local government spending).[10]

Medicaid was enacted in 1965 as part of the same law that created the Medicare program (the Social Security Amendments of 1965; P.L. 89-97). Medicaid was designed to provide coverage to groups with a wide range of health care needs that historically were excluded from the private health insurance market (e.g., individuals with disabilities who require LTSS or indigent populations in geographic locations where access to providers is limited). Because of the diversity of the populations that Medicaid serves, Medicaid offers some benefits that typically are not covered by major insurance plans offered in the private market (e.g., institutional and home

---

[4] The *health care safety net* consists of those organizations and programs, in both the public and private sectors, with a legal obligation or a commitment to provide direct health care services to uninsured and underinsured populations.

[5] U.S. Census Bureau, American Community Survey Tables for Health Insurance Coverage, Table HI-05, Health Insurance Coverage Status and Type of Coverage by State and Age for All People: 2017.

[6] U.S. Census Bureau, 2017 American Community Survey 1-Year Estimates, "Public Health Insurance Coverage by Type and Selected Characteristics," Table S2704.

[7] Henry J. Kaiser Family Foundation, *Health Insurance Coverage of the Nonelderly (0-64) with Incomes below 100% Federal Poverty Level (FPL)*, State Health Facts, at https://www.kff.org/other/state-indicator, accessed March 8, 2019.

[8] Based on CRS analysis of National Health Expenditure Account (NHEA) data obtained from CMS, Office of the Actuary, prepared November 2018.

[9] Joyce A. Martin, Brady E. Hamilton, and Michelle J. K. Osterman, et al., *Births: Final Data for 2017*, National Center for Health Statistics, National Vital Statistics Reports, vol. 67, no.8, November 7, 2018.

[10] Kinsey Hasstedt, Adam Sonfield, and Rachel Benson Gold, *Public Funding for Family Planning and Abortion Services, FY1980-2015*, Guttmacher Institute, April 2017.

and community-based LTSS or early and periodic screening, diagnosis, and treatment [EPSDT] services).

Medicaid also pays for Medicare premiums and/or cost sharing for low-income seniors and individuals with disabilities, who are eligible for both programs and referred to as *dual-eligible beneficiaries*. For other Medicaid enrollees, cost sharing (e.g., premiums and co-payments) generally are nominal, which may not be the case with coverage available through the private health insurance market. The Medicaid program pays for services provided by special classes of providers, such as federally qualified health centers (FQHCs), rural health clinics (RHCs), and Indian Health Service (IHS) facilities that provide health care services to populations in areas where access to traditional physician care may be limited.

This chapter describes the basic elements of Medicaid, focusing on who is eligible, what services are covered, how enrollees share in the cost of care, how the program is financed. The report also explains waivers, provider payments, and program integrity activities. At the end of the report is a section with additional Medicaid resources.

ELIGIBILITY

Eligibility for Medicaid is determined by both federal and state law, whereby states set individual eligibility criteria within federal minimum standards. As a result, there is substantial variability in Medicaid eligibility across states. Therefore, the ways that an individual might qualify for Medicaid are largely reflective of state policy decisions within broad federal requirements.

In general, individuals qualify for Medicaid coverage by meeting the requirements of a specific eligibility pathway offered by the state. Some eligibility pathways are mandatory, meaning all states with a Medicaid program must cover them; others are optional. Within this framework, states are afforded discretion in determining certain eligibility criteria for both mandatory and optional eligibility groups. In addition, states may apply to the Centers for Medicare & Medicaid Services (CMS) for a waiver of federal law to expand health coverage beyond the mandatory and optional eligibility groups specified in federal statute (see the "Medicaid Program Waivers" section for more information).

An eligibility pathway is the federal statutory reference(s) under Title XIX of the Social Security Act (SSA) that extends Medicaid coverage to one or more groups of individuals.[11] Each eligibility pathway specifies the group of individuals covered by the pathway (i.e., *categorical criteria*), the financial requirements applicable to the group (i.e., *financial criteria*),[12] whether the pathway is mandatory or optional, and the extent of the state's discretion over the pathway's requirements. Individuals in need of Medicaid-covered LTSS must demonstrate the need for long-term care by meeting state-based eligibility criteria for services, and they also may be subject to a separate set of Medicaid financial eligibility rules in order to receive LTSS coverage. All Medicaid applicants regardless of their eligibility pathway must meet federal and state requirements regarding residency, immigration status, and documentation of U.S. citizenship.[13]

Often an applicant's eligibility pathway dictates the Medicaid state plan services that a given program enrollee is entitled to (e.g., women eligible due to their pregnancy status are entitled to Medicaid pregnancy-related services). When applying to Medicaid, an individual may be eligible for the program through more than one pathway. In this situation, an individual is generally permitted to choose the pathway that would be most beneficial in terms of the treatment of income and sometimes assets

---

[11] Although most eligibility pathways are specified in Title XIX of the Social Security Act (SSA), some pathways are specified in other parts of the SSA, in other federal laws, or in regulations prescribed by CMS pursuant to authority provided in the SSA. See SSA §1939.

[12] Some groups, such as young people under the age of 26 who have aged out of foster care and individuals eligible through the breast and cervical cancer treatment pathway, are eligible for Medicaid coverage without regard to income and assets.

[13] Federal Medicaid residency requirements can be found at SSA §§1902(a)(16), 1902(a) and 1902(b)(2). Federal Medicaid eligibility requirements for non-citizens generally can be found at SSA §§401, 402(b), 403, 1137, and §421 of the Personal Responsibility and Work Opportunity Reconciliation Act (PRWORA; P.L. 104-193). Federal Medicaid citizenship documentation requirements can be found at SSA §§1902(a)(46), 1902(ee), 1903(x), and 1903(a)(3)(H).

when determining Medicaid eligibility, but also in terms of the available benefits associated with each eligibility pathway.

Medicaid eligibility determinations generally apply for 12 months before an eligibility redetermination must occur. Individuals may be retroactively eligible for Medicaid up to three months prior to the month of application, if the individual received covered services and would have been eligible had he or she applied during that period.[14]

The following sections describe Medicaid's categorical and financial eligibility criteria as well as additional eligibility requirements for Medicaid covered-LTSS.

Categorical Eligibility

Medicaid categorical eligibility criteria are the characteristics that define the population qualifying for Medicaid coverage under a particular eligibility pathway; in other words, the nonfinancial requirements that an individual must meet to be considered eligible under an eligibility group. Medicaid covers several broad coverage groups, including children, pregnant women, adults, individuals with disabilities, and individuals 65 years of age and older (i.e., aged). There are a number of distinct Medicaid eligibility pathways within each of these broad coverage groups.

Historically, Medicaid eligibility was limited to poor families with dependent children who received cash assistance under the former Aid to Families with Dependent Children (AFDC) program, as well as poor aged, blind, or disabled individuals who received cash assistance under the Supplemental Security Income (SSI) program. Medicaid eligibility rules reflected these historical program linkages both in terms of the categories of individuals who were served and in that the financial eligibility rules were generally based on the most closely related social program for the group involved (e.g., AFDC program rules for low-income families with dependentchildren and pregnant women, and SSI program rules for aged,

[14] SSA §1902(a)(34); 42 C.F.R. §435.916.

blind, or disabled).[15] Over time, Medicaid eligibility has expanded to allow states to extend Medicaid coverage to individuals beyond those who were eligible based on receipt of cash assistance, including the most recent addition of the ACA Medicaid expansion population (i.e., nonelderly adults with income up to 133% of FPL).[16] Medicaid's financial eligibility rules also have been modified over time for certain groups.[17]

If a state participates in Medicaid, the following are examples of eligibility groups that *must* be provided Medicaid coverage:

- certain low-income families, including parents, that meet the financial requirements of the former AFDC cash assistance program;
- pregnant women with annual income at or below 133% of FPL;
- children with family income at or below 133% of FPL;
- aged, blind, or disabled individuals who receive cash assistance under the SSI program;[18]
- children receiving foster care, adoption assistance, or kinship guardianship assistance under SSA Title IV–E;
- certain former foster care youth;[19]

---

[15] 42 C.F.R. §435.601.

[16] The poverty guidelines (also referred to as the federal poverty level) are issued each year in the *Federal Register* by HHS. The guidelines, which are a simplification of the U.S. Census Bureau's poverty thresholds, are used for administrative purposes—for instance, determining financial eligibility for certain federal programs. The 2019 poverty guidelines for an individual are $12,490 in the 48 contiguous states; $15,600 in Alaska; and $14,380 in Hawaii. For more information, see https://aspe.hhs.gov/poverty-guidelines.

[17] For more information, see CRS Report R43861, The Use of Modified Adjusted Gross Income (MAGI) in Federal Health Programs.

[18] For SSI recipients, states have the option to use certain eligibility criteria for Medicaid that are more restrictive than SSI but no more restrictive than those criteria in effect on January 1, 1972. In these states, SSI receipt does not automatically extend Medicaid eligibility. States that use this alternative to SSI program rules typically are referred to as *209(b) states*, which is the section of the Social Security Amendments of 1972 (SSA 72; P.L. 92-603) that provided this authority. In 2019, eight states provide Medicaid to SSI recipients using this method: Connecticut, Hawaii, Illinois, Minnesota, Missouri, New Hampshire, North Dakota, and Virginia.

[19] For more information, see CRS In Focus IF11010, Medicaid Coverage for Former Foster Youth Up to Age 26.

- individuals eligible for the Qualified Medicare Beneficiary program;[20] and
- certain groups of legal permanent resident immigrants.[21]

Examples of eligibility groups to which states *may* provide Medicaid include the following:

- pregnant women with annual income between 133% and 185% of FPL;
- infants with family income between 133% and 185% of FPL;
- certain individuals who require institutional care and have incomes up to 300% of the SSI federal benefit rate;
- certain *medically needy* individuals (e.g., children, pregnant women, aged, blind, or disabled) who are otherwise eligible for Medicaid but who have incomes too high to qualify and spend down their income on medical care;[22] and
- nonelderly adults with income at or below 133% of FPL (i.e., the ACA Medicaid expansion).[23]

Some individuals who are eligible for Medicaid are also eligible for Medicare. Individuals enrolled in both Medicaid and Medicare are referred to as *dual-eligible individuals*. For more information about this population, see the textbox entitled "Dual-Eligible Beneficiaries."

---

[20] Under the Qualified Medicare Beneficiary (QMB) program, Medicaid helps pay premiums, deductibles, coinsurance, and co-payments for Medicare Part A, Medicare Part B, or both for dual-eligible individuals (i.e., individuals eligible for both Medicare and Medicaid) with annual income less than 100% of the federal poverty level.

[21] These groups also must meet all other Medicaid eligibility requirements and include refugees for the first seven years after entry into the United States; asylees for the first seven years after asylum is granted; lawful permanent aliens with 40 quarters of creditable coverage under Social Security; and immigrants who are honorably discharged U.S. military veterans.

[22] For these groups, individuals may qualify for Medicaid by meeting the medically needy income standard or spend down to the medically needy income standard by incurring and paying for medical expenses.

[23] For more information about the ACA Medicaid expansion, see CRS In Focus IF10399, *Overview of the ACA Medicaid Expansion*.

Dual-Eligible Beneficiaries

In CY2013, there were 10.7 million dual-eligible beneficiaries (individuals enrolled in both Medicare and Medicaid), which was 14.5% of Medicaid enrollment.[24] Although commonly addressed as a single population, dual-eligible beneficiaries are diverse. While dual-eligible beneficiaries tend to be sicker and poorer than the Medicaid population as a whole, not all dual-eligible beneficiaries are in poor health.

There are numerous Medicaid eligibility pathways for dual-eligible beneficiaries with different types of Medicaid coverage, but the two main categories of dual-eligible individuals are full dual-eligible beneficiaries and partial dual-eligible beneficiaries. Full dual-eligible beneficiaries receive full benefits from Medicare, and Medicaid provides them with full benefits in addition to financial assistance with their Medicare premiums and cost sharing. Partial dual-eligible beneficiaries receive full benefits from Medicare and financial assistance from Medicaid for Medicare premiums and cost sharing. In CY2013, there were 7.7 million full duals, with Medicaid spending totaling $116.8 billion, and 3.0 million partial duals, with $2.1 billion in Medicaid spending.[25]

Financial Eligibility

Medicaid is also a means-tested program that is limited to those with financial need. However, the criteria used to determine financial eligibility—income and sometimes resource (i.e., asset) tests—vary by eligibility group.

For most eligibility groups the criteria used to determine eligibility are based on modified adjusted gross income (MAGI) income counting rules. There is no resource or asset test used to determine Medicaid financial eligibility for MAGI-eligible individuals.[26]

---

[24] Medicare Payment Advisory Commission and the Medicaid and CHIP Payment and Access Commission (MACPAC), *Beneficiaries Dually Eligible for Medicare and Medicaid*, Data Book, January 2018.

[25] Ibid.

[26] In addition, for some groups such as former foster care youth who aged out of foster care, no income eligibility test is applied. For more information on the use of modified adjusted

While MAGI applies to most Medicaid-eligible populations, certain populations such as older adults and individuals with disabilities are statutorily exempt from MAGI income counting rules. Instead, Medicaid financial eligibility for MAGI-exempted populations is based on the income counting rules that match the most closely related social program for the group involved (e.g., SSI program rules for aged, blind, or disabled eligibility groups). For MAGI-exempt eligibility groups, income disregards and assets or resource tests may apply.

Additional Eligibility Requirements for LTSS Coverage

Medicaid enrollees, many of whom qualify based on aged or disabled categorical criteria, may also have long-term care needs. In general, individuals in need of Medicaid-covered LTSS must also meet state-based functional and/or disease or condition-specific eligibility criteria. In other words, they must demonstrate the need for long-term care. There are certain pathways that establish eligibility to Medicaid-covered LTSS either for individuals receiving institutional care or for those who need the level of care provided in an institution and receive Medicaid-covered home and community-based services (HCBS).[27] Most states offer HCBS under waiver programs that operate outside of Medicaid state plan requirements (see the "Medicaid Program Waivers" section for more information).

Applicants seeking certain Medicaid-covered LTSS are also subject to a separate set of Medicaid financial eligibility rules in order to receive such services (e.g., limits on the value of home equity, asset transfer rules). These additional financial rules attempt to ensure that program applicants

---

gross income (MAGI) as well as MAGI-exempt groups, see CRS Report R43861, *The Use of Modified Adjusted Gross Income (MAGI) in Federal Health Programs*.

[27] There are certain optional eligibility pathways for older adults and individuals with disabilities—Special Income Level, Special Home and Community-Based Waiver Group, Home and Community-Based Services (HCBS) State Plan, and Katie Beckett—that establish eligibility to Medicaid-covered long-term services and supports (LTSS) either for individuals receiving institutional care or those who need the level of care provided in an institution and receive Medicaid-covered HCBS.

apply their assets toward the cost of their care and do not divest them to gain eligibility sooner than would occur otherwise.

In addition, Medicaid specifies rules for equitably allocating income and assets to non-Medicaidcovered spouses for the purposes of determining LTSS coverage eligibility for nursing facility services and some HCBS. Commonly referred to as spousal impoverishment rules, these rules are intended to prevent the impoverishment of the spouse who does not need LTSS.[28]

Medicaid Enrollment

Figure 1 shows historical and projected Medicaid enrollment for FY2000 through FY2026. The figure shows steady enrollment growth, especially among nondisabled children and adults as a result of the recessions in the early and late 2000s.[29] During periods of economic downturn, Medicaid programs face enrollment increases at a faster rate because job and income losses make more people eligible.

Since the implementation of the ACA Medicaid expansion in 2014, most of the growth in Medicaid enrollment is attributed to the expansion. Excluding the expansion adults, Medicaid enrollment was relatively flat due to low unemployment rates over the past couple years.[30] For FY2017 through FY2026, the aged population is projected to be the fastest-growing Medicaid population due to baby boomers reaching the age of 65.[31]

---

[28] Historically, these rules have applied to the spouse of participants receiving institutional care. However, under ACA Section 2404, these rules were extended for a limited time to the spouse of participants receiving certain home and community-based services and are scheduled to sunset on September 30, 2019. CRS Report R43506, *Medicaid Financial Eligibility for Long-Term Services and Supports*.

[29] According to the National Bureau of Economic Research, the United States was in recession from March 2001 through November 2001 and December 2007 through June 2009. See https://www.nber.org/cycles.html.

[30] Medicaid enrollment grew at 0.2% and 0.3% in FY2016 and FY2017, respectively. (Christopher J. Truffer, Christian J. Wolfe, and Kathryn E. Rennie, *2017 Actuarial Report on the Financial Outlook for Medicaid*, Office of the Actuary, CMS, HHS, 2018.)

[31] Christopher J. Truffer, Christian J. Wolfe, and Kathryn E. Rennie, *2017 Actuarial Report on the Financial Outlook for Medicaid*, Office of the Actuary, CMS, HHS, 2018.

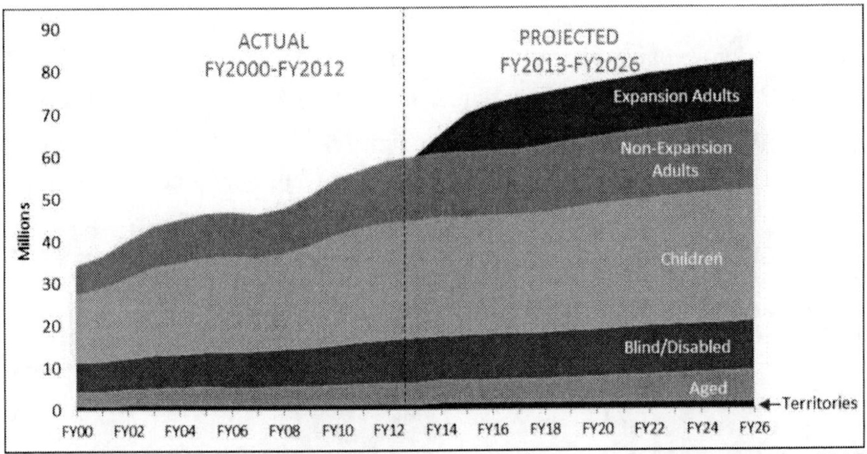

Source: Christopher J. Truffer, Christian J. Wolfe, and Kathryn E. Rennie, 2017 Actuarial Report on the Financial Outlook for Medicaid, Office of the Actuary, Centers for Medicare & Medicaid Services (CMS), U.S. Department of Health & Human Services (HHS), 2018.

Notes: Enrollment is measured by person-year equivalents, which is the average enrollment over the course of the year.

For purposes of this figure, Expansion Adults are adult enrollees who are newly eligible in 2014 and later as a result of the expanded eligibility criteria in the Patient Protection and Affordable Care Act (ACA; 111-148, as amended). Other eligible adults who become enrolled as a result of the publicity and outreach efforts associated with the ACA are included with Non-Expansion Adults, and their dependent children are included with Children in this figure.

Figure 1. Past and Projected Medicaid Enrollment, by Population. (FY2000–FY2026)

Share of Enrollment Versus Expenditures, by Population

Different Medicaid enrollment groups have very different service utilization patterns. Larger enrollment groups account for a smaller proportion of Medicaid expenditures, while some smaller enrollment groups are responsible for a larger proportion of Medicaid expenditures.

As shown in *Figure 2*, for FY2016, together Medicaid enrollment for children, non-expansion adults, and expansion adults comprised 77% of Medicaid enrollment but accounted for only 46% of Medicaid's total benefit spending. In contrast, together the disabled and aged populations represented about 23% of Medicaid enrollment but accounted for a larger share of Medicaid benefit spending (54%). While these statistics vary somewhat from year to year and state to state, the patterns described above generally hold true across years.

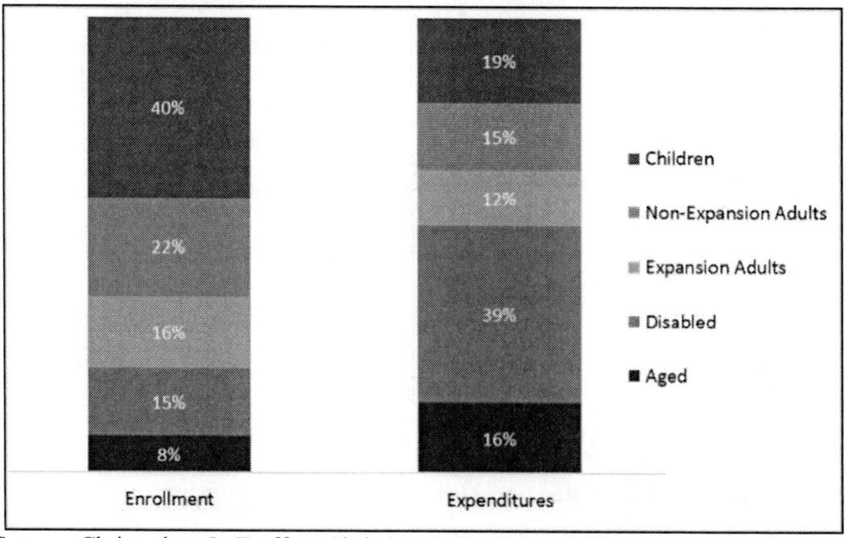

Source: Christopher J. Truffer, Christian J. Wolfe, and Kathryn E. Rennie, 2017 Actuarial Report on the Financial Outlook for Medicaid, Office of the Actuary, CMS, HHS, 2018.

Notes: Totals and components exclude disproportionate share hospital expenditures (i.e., payments to hospitals treating large numbers of low-income patients), territory enrollees and expenditures, and other adjustments. May not sum to totals due to rounding.

Figure 2. Estimated Medicaid Enrollment and Expenditures for Benefits, by Enrollment Group as a Share of Total. (FY2016)

BENEFITS

Medicaid coverage includes a wide variety of preventive, primary, and acute care services as well as LTSS.[32] Not everyone enrolled in Medicaid has access to the same set of services. An enrollee's eligibility pathway determines the available services within a benefit package. Federal law provides two primary benefit packages for state Medicaid programs: (1) traditional benefits and (2) alternative benefit plans (ABPs). Each of these packages is summarized in *Table 1*. For the medically needy subgroup, states may offer a more restrictive benefit package than is available to other enrollees. In addition, states can use waiver authority (e.g., SSA Section 1115) to tailor benefit packages to specified Medicaid subgroups as well as offer services outside traditional or ABP coverage, such as LTSS (see "Medicaid Program Waivers" for more information about Section 1115 waivers).

In general, when Medicaid enrollees have other sources of insurance/payment (including Medicare), Medicaid is the payer of last resort. States can provide Medicaid coverage to individuals whose existing health insurance is limited (sometimes referred to as underinsured). In these cases, Medicaid wraps around that coverage (i.e., additional coverage for services covered under Medicaid but not under the other source of coverage).[33]

The following sections summarize Medicaid traditional benefits and ABPs. Then, there is a section comparing benefits included in traditional Medicaid coverage and those that are commonly included in ABPs.

---

[32] LTSS benefits are available in institutional and home and community-based (HCBS) settings, and they include nursing facility services, home health, case management services, personal care services, and private duty nursing, among others.

[33] For related details, see federal regulations at 42 C.F.R. 433.135, 433.138, and 433.152.

Table 1. Examples of Medicaid Mandatory and Optional Benefits for Traditional Benefits and Alternative Benefit Plans (ABPs)

Type of Benefit	Traditional Benefits	ABPs
Mandatory	• Inpatient hospital services • EPSDT (< the age of 21) • Nursing facility care (aged 21+) • Physician services • FQHC services • Family planning services • Pregnancy-related services • Home health	• Hospitalization services • EPSDT (< the age of 21) • Preventive services • Prescription drugs • FQHC services • Family planning services • Maternity and newborn care • Rehabilitative services • Mental health and substance use disorder services
Optional	• Clinic services • Prescription drugs • Physical, occupational, and speech therapy services • Dental services for adults • Personal care	For special-needs subgroups, option to receive traditional benefits or enroll in an ABP plan.

Sources: Title XIX of the Social Security Act and related federal guidance. Notes: ABP = Alternative benefit plan; EPSDT = Early and periodic screening, diagnostic, and treatment services; FQHC = Federally qualified health center.

Traditional Medicaid Benefits

Traditional Medicaid benefits include primary and acute care as well as LTSS. The traditional Medicaid program requires states to cover a wide array of mandatory services (e.g., inpatient hospital care, lab and x-ray services, physician care, nursing facility services for individuals aged 21 and older). In addition, states may provide optional services, some of which commonly are covered (e.g., personal care services, prescription drugs, clinic services, physical therapy, and prosthetic devices).

States define the specific features of each covered benefit within four broad federal guidelines:

- Each service must be *sufficient in amount*, *duration*, and *scope* to reasonably achieve its purpose. States may place appropriate limits on a service based on such criteria as medical necessity.
- Within a state, services available to the various population groups must be equal in amount, duration, and scope. This requirement is the *comparability rule*.
- With certain exceptions, the amount, duration, and scope of benefits must be the same statewide, referred to as the *statewideness rule*.
- With certain exceptions, enrollees must have *freedom of choice* among health care providers or managed care entities participating in Medicaid. (See "Service Delivery Systems" for information about managed care.)

The breadth of coverage for a given benefit can, and does, vary from state to state, even for mandatory services. For example, states may place different limits on the amount of inpatient hospital services a beneficiary can receive in a year (e.g., up to 15 inpatient days per year in one state versus unlimited inpatient days in another state)—as long as applicable requirements are met regarding sufficiency of amount, duration, and scope; comparability; statewideness; and freedom of choice. Exceptions to state limits may be permitted under circumstances defined by the state.

Alternative Benefit Plans

As an alternative to providing all the mandatory and selected optional benefits under traditional Medicaid, the Deficit Reduction Act of 2005 (DRA; P.L. 109-171) gave states the option to enroll state-specified groups in what was referred to as benchmark or benchmark-equivalent coverage but currently are called alternative benefit plans (ABPs).[34] Under ABPs, states must provide comprehensive benefit coverage that is based on a

[34] For more information on Medicaid Alternative Benefit Plan Coverage, see CRS Report R45412, *Medicaid Alternative Benefit Plan Coverage: Frequently Asked Questions*.

coverage benchmark rather than a list of discrete items and services as under traditional Medicaid.

ABPs must qualify as either benchmark or benchmark-equivalent coverage. Under benchmark coverage, ABP benefits are at least equal to one of the statutorily specified benchmark plans (i.e., one of three commercial health insurance products, or a fourth "Secretary-approved" coverage option).[35] Under benchmark-equivalent coverage, ABP benefits include certain specified services and the overall benefits are at least actuarially equivalent to one of the statutorily specified benchmark coverage packages.

Unlike traditional Medicaid benefit coverage, coverage under an ABP must include at least the essential health benefits (EHBs) that most plans in the private health insurance market are required to furnish.[36] In addition, ABPs must include a variety of specific services, including services under Medicaid's early and periodic screening, diagnostic, and testing (EPSDT) benefit; family planning services and supplies; and both emergency and nonemergency transportation to and from providers. In general, the EHBs do not include LTSS. However, states may choose to include LTSS in their ABPs.

Under ABPs, states are permitted to waive the statewideness and comparability requirements that apply to traditional Medicaid benefits. This flexibility permits the state to define populations that are served and the specific benefit packages that apply. However, states that choose to implement the ACA Medicaid expansion are required to provide ABP coverage to the individuals eligible for Medicaid through the expansion

---

[35] The three ABP benchmark commercial insurance products include (1) the standard Blue Cross/Blue Shield preferred provider option service plan offered through the Federal Employees Health Benefit Program-equivalent health insurance coverage; (2) the health benefits coverage plan offered to state employees; and (3) the commercial health maintenance organization with the largest insured commercial, non-Medicaid enrollment in the state.

[36] The 10 essential health benefits required under the ACA include (1) ambulatory patient services, (2) emergency services, (3) hospitalization, (4) maternity and newborn care, (5) mental health and substance use disorder services (including behavioral health treatment), (6) prescription drugs, (7) rehabilitative and habilitative services and devices, (8) laboratory services, (9) preventive and wellness services and chronic disease management, and (10) pediatric services, including oral and vision care. For more information about EHBs, see CRS In Focus IF10287, *The Essential Health Benefits (EHB).*

(with exceptions for selected special-needs subgroups). Specific populations are exempt from mandatory enrollment in ABPs (e.g., those with special health care needs such as disabling mental disorders or serious and complex medical conditions). These individuals must be offered the option of a benefit plan that includes traditional Medicaid state plan services, which may include LTSS.

Comparing Traditional Medicaid Benefits to ABPs

It is difficult to draw comparisons about the ways in which traditional Medicaid benefits are similar to and different from ABP benefits, because the scope of each type of benefit package varies from state to state. This variability is largely a reflection of state choices in covering optional benefits, in addition to the mandatory Medicaid state plan benefits, as well as state choices for the base-benchmark for the EHBs that must be covered under ABPs.

However, differences in the federal laws regarding the scope of required benefits under traditional Medicaid and those required under ABPs highlight some common differences between the two types of benefits packages. For example, care in a nursing facility for individuals over the age of 21 is a required benefit under traditional Medicaid, whereas nursing home care is not a required benefit under ABPs.

Conversely, rehabilitative and habilitative services and devices, preventive and wellness services, and mental health and substance use disorder services are all required benefits under ABPs. By contrast, these APB benefit categories do not correspond to specific benefit categories under traditional Medicaid. Rather, services in these benefit categories could be covered under different benefit categories, such as physician services or physical, occupational, and speech therapy services.

To further illustrate this point, *behavioral health* (or any similar term) is not explicitly included among the required benefit categories under traditional Medicaid. Instead, most types of behavioral health benefits (e.g., the services of clinical psychologists and licensed clinical social workers and prescription drugs) are optional. By contrast, behavioral health benefits are mandatory under ABPs because "mental health and substance use disorder services, including behavioral health treatment" are included among the EHBs.

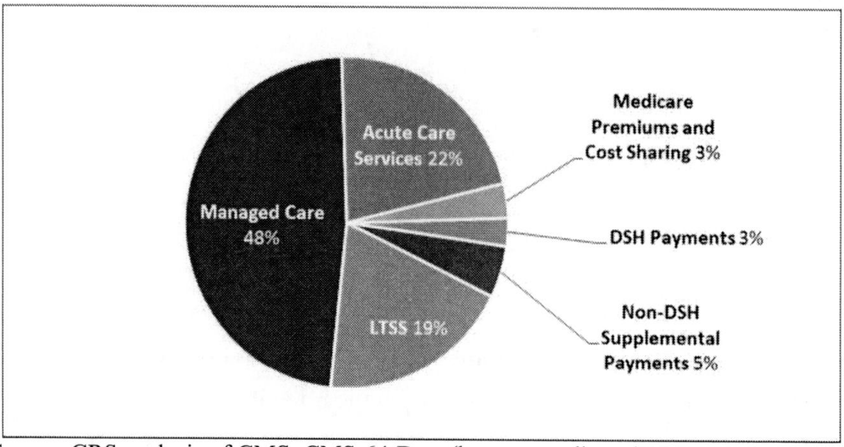

Source: CRS analysis of CMS, CMS-64 Data (base expenditures), FY2018 as of April 29, 2019.

Notes: Medical assistance expenditures exclude Medicaid expenditures for administrative activities. Managed care includes capitated payments under which Medicaid enrollees get most or all of their services through an organization under contract with the state (see "Service Delivery Systems" for information about managed care). Supplemental payments are Medicaid payments made to providers that are separate from and in addition to the standard payment rates for services rendered to Medicaid enrollees, and disproportionate share hospital (DSH) payments are one type of supplemental payments. Acute care services include prescription drugs.

DSH = Disproportionate share hospital LTSS = Long-term services and supports

Figure 3. Medicaid Medical Assistance Expenditures, by Service Category. (FY2018)

Medicaid Service Spending

Figure 3 below shows the nationwide distribution of Medicaid expenditures across broad categories of service for FY2017. These data illustrate that 49% of benefit spending was for capitated payments under managed care arrangements (see "Service Delivery Systems" for information about managed care). The remaining 51% of benefit spending was FFS, and FFS spending on LTSS and acute care services accounted for 21% and 20%, respectively, of Medicaid benefit spending.

BENEFICIARY COST SHARING

Federal statutes and regulations address the circumstances under which enrollees may share in the costs of Medicaid, both in terms of participation-related cost sharing (e.g., monthly premiums) and point-of-service cost sharing (e.g., co-payments [i.e., flat dollar amounts paid directly to providers for services rendered]).[37] States can require certain beneficiaries to share in the cost of Medicaid services, but there are limits on (1) the amounts that states can impose, (2) the beneficiary groups that can be required to pay, and (3) the services for which cost sharing can be charged.[38]

In general, premiums and enrollment fees often are prohibited. However, premiums may be imposed on certain enrollees, such as individuals with incomes above 150% of FPL, certain working individuals with disabilities, and certain children with disabilities.

States can impose cost sharing at the point of service, such as co-payments,[39] coinsurance,[40] deductibles,[41] and other similar charges, on most Medicaid-covered benefits up to federal limits that vary by income. Some subgroups of beneficiaries are exempt from cost sharing (e.g., children under 18 years of age and pregnant women).

---

[37] For more information about Medicaid cost sharing, see CRS Report R43850, *Out-of-Pocket Costs for Medicaid Beneficiaries: In Brief.*

[38] For more information about these limits, see CMS, *Cost Sharing Out of Pocket Costs*, at https://www.medicaid.gov/ medicaid/cost-sharing/out-of-pocket-costs/index.html.

[39] A *co-payment* is a specified dollar amount for each item or service delivered.

[40] *Coinsurance* is a specified percentage of the cost or charge for a specific service delivered.

[41] A *deductible* is a specified dollar amount paid for certain services rendered during a specific time period (e.g., per month or quarter) before health coverage (e.g., Medicaid) begins to pay for care.

The aggregate cap on participation-related cost sharing (e.g., monthly premiums) and point-ofservice cost sharing (e.g., co-payments) is generally up to 5% of monthly or quarterly household income.[42]

In addition, beneficiaries receiving certain Medicaid-covered LTSS are required to apply their income exceeding specified amounts toward the cost of their care. These reductions from a beneficiary's income are referred to as *post-eligibility treatment of income* and are not subject to the 5% aggregate cost-sharing cap described above.[43] The amounts a beneficiary may retain for their personal use vary by care setting (i.e., nursing facility versus home and community-based).

SERVICE DELIVERY SYSTEMS

In general, most benefits for to Medicaid enrollees are delivered and paid for via two service delivery systems: *fee-for-service* (FFS) or *managed care*. Under the FFS delivery system, health care providers are paid by the state Medicaid program for each service provided to a Medicaid enrollee. Under the managed care delivery system, Medicaid enrollees get most or all of their services through an organization under contract with the state.

States traditionally have used the FFS service delivery model for Medicaid, but since the 1990s, the share of Medicaid enrollees covered by the managed care model has increased dramatically. Initially, states used managed care to deliver health care services to the healthiest Medicaid populations, including children and parents. However, recently, more states are turning to managed care for their aged and disabled populations.

There are three main types of Medicaid managed care:

- *Comprehensive risk-based managed care*—states contract with managed care organizations (MCOs) to provide a comprehensive

---

[42] SSA §1916A.

[43] For further information on these Post-Eligibility Treatment of Income rules, see CRS Report R43506, *Medicaid Financial Eligibility for Long-Term Services and Supports*.

package of benefits to certain Medicaid enrollees. States usually pay the MCOs on a capitated basis, which means the states prospectively pay the MCOs a fixed monthly rate per enrollee to provide or arrange for most health care services. MCOs then pay providers for services to enrollees.

- *Primary care case management (PCCM)*—states contract with primary care providers to provide case management services to Medicaid enrollees. Typically, under PCCM, the primary care provider receives a monthly case management fee per enrollee for coordination of care, but the provider continues to receive fee-for-service payments for the medical care services utilized by Medicaid enrollees.
- *Limited benefit plans*—these plans look like MCOs in that states usually contract with a plan and pay it on a capitated basis. The difference is that limited benefit plans provide only one or two Medicaid services (e.g., behavioral health or dental services).

As of July 1, 2017, about 82% of Medicaid enrollees were covered by some form of managed care.[44] Two states (South Carolina and Washington) covered all Medicaid enrollees under managed care, and two states (Alaska and Connecticut) did not have any managed care coverage. The rest of the states use some combination of managed care and FFS coverage.[45]

The most prevalent type of managed care is the comprehensive risk-based managed care that is provided through MCOs, with 69% of Medicaid enrollees with comprehensive risk-based managed care as of July 1, 2017.[46] States' use of comprehensive risk-based managed care varies significantly, as shown in *Figure 4*.

---

[44] This figure excludes Medicaid enrollment in the territories. (CMS, *Medicaid Managed Care Enrollment and Program Characteristics, 2017,* Table 4, Winter 2019.)

[45] Ibid.

[46] This figure excludes Medicaid enrollment in the territories. (CMS, *Medicaid Managed Care Enrollment and Program Characteristics, 2017,* Table 4, Winter 2019.)

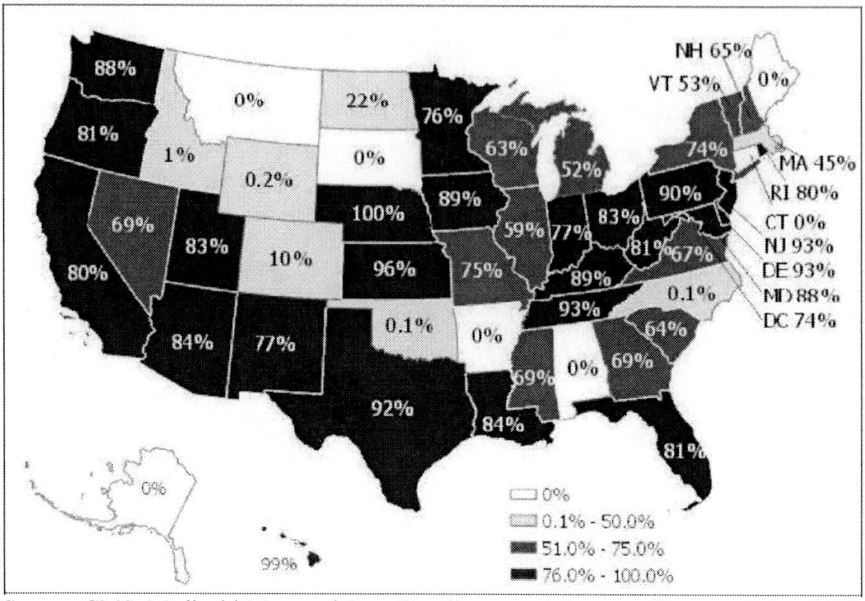

Source: CMS, Medicaid Managed Care Enrollment and Program Characteristics, 2017, Table 4, Winter 2019.

Notes: Medicaid enrollment in comprehensive managed care represents an unduplicated count of Medicaid beneficiaries enrolled in a managed care plan that provides comprehensive benefits (acute, primary care, specialty, and any other), as well as Programs for All-Inclusive Care for the Elderly (PACE). It excludes enrollees who are enrolled in a Financial Alignment Initiative Medicare-Medicaid Plan as their only form of managed care.

Figure 4. Percentage of Medicaid Enrollees with Comprehensive Risk-Based Managed Care, by State. (As of July 1, 2017)

FINANCING

The federal government and the states jointly finance Medicaid.[47] The federal government reimburses states for a portion (i.e., the federal share) of each state's Medicaid program costs. Because federal Medicaid funding is an open-ended entitlement to states, there is no upper limit or cap on the

[47] For more information about Medicaid financing and expenditures, see CRS Report R42640, *Medicaid Financing and Expenditures*.

amount of federal Medicaid funds a state may receive. In FY2018, Medicaid expenditures totaled $616 billion. The federal share totaled $386 billion and the state share was $230 billion.[48]

Federal Share

The federal government's share of most Medicaid expenditures is established by the federal medical assistance percentage (FMAP) rate, which generally is determined annually and varies by state according to each state's per capita income relative to the U.S. per capita income.[49] The formula provides higher FMAP rates, or federal reimbursement rates, to states with lower per capita incomes, and it provides lower FMAP rates to states with higher per capita incomes.

FMAP rates have a statutory minimum of 50% and a statutory maximum of 83%.[50] For a state with an FMAP of 60%, the state gets 60 cents back from the federal government for every dollar the state spends on its Medicaid program. In FY2019, FMAP rates range from 50% (14 states) to 76% (Mississippi).

The FMAP rate is used to reimburse states for the federal share of most Medicaid expenditures, but exceptions to the regular FMAP rate have been made for certain states (e.g., the District of Columbia and the territories), situations (e.g., during economic downturns), populations (e.g., the ACA Medicaid expansion population and certain women with breast or cervical cancer), providers (e.g., Indian Health Service facilities), and services (e.g., family planning and home health services). In addition, the federal share for most Medicaid administrative costs does not vary by state and is generally 50%.

While most federal Medicaid funding is provided on an open-ended basis, certain types of federal Medicaid funding are capped. For instance,

[48] CMS, CMS-64 data as of April 29, 2019.

[49] For more detail about the federal medical assistance percentage (FMAP) rate, see CRS Report R42640, *Medicaid Financing and Expenditures*.

[50] SSA §1905(b).

federal disproportionate share hospital (DSH)[51] funding to states cannot exceed a state-specific annual allotment. Also, Medicaid programs in the territories (i.e., American Samoa, Guam, Northern Mariana Islands, Puerto Rico, and the Virgin Islands) are subject to annual spending caps.[52]

State Share

The federal government provides broad guidelines to states regarding allowable funding sources for the *state share* (also referred to as the *nonfederal share*) of Medicaid expenditures. However, to a large extent, states are free to determine how to fund their share of Medicaid expenditures. As a result, there is significant variation from state to state in funding sources.

States can use state general funds (i.e., personal income, sales, and corporate income taxes) and other state funds (e.g., provider taxes,[53] local government funds, tobacco settlement funds, etc.) to finance the state share of Medicaid. Federal statute allows as much as 60% of the state share to come from local government funding.[54] Federal regulations also stipulate that the state share not be funded with federal funds (Medicaid or otherwise).[55] In state fiscal year 2017, on average, 72% of the state share of Medicaid expenditures was financed by state general funds, and the remaining 28% was financed by other state funds.[56]

---

[51] For more information about Medicaid DSH payments, see CRS Report R42865, *Medicaid Disproportionate Share Hospital Payments*.

[52] For more information about Medicaid funding for the territories, see CRS In Focus IF11012, *Medicaid Funding for the Territories*.

[53] States are able to use revenues from health care provider taxes to help finance their share of Medicaid expenditures as long as the provider tax is broad-based and uniform. For more information about provider taxes, see CRS Report RS22843, *Medicaid Provider Taxes*.

[54] SSA §1902(a)(2).

[55] 42 C.F.R. 433.51(c).

[56] National Association of State Budget Officers, *2018 State Expenditure Report: Fiscal Years 2016-2018,* 2018.

Expenditures

The cost of Medicaid, like most health expenditures, historically increased at a rate significantly faster than the overall rate of U.S. economic growth, as measured by gross domestic product. In the past, much of Medicaid's expenditure growth has been due to federal or state expansions of Medicaid eligibility criteria, such as the ACA Medicaid expansion.

Medicaid expenditures are influenced by economic, demographic, and programmatic factors. Economic factors include health care prices, unemployment rates (see the "Medicaid Enrollment" section for a discussion of the impact of the unemployment rate on Medicaid enrollment, which also impacts expenditures), and individuals' wages. Demographic factors include population growth and the age distribution of the population. Programmatic factors include state decisions regarding optional eligibility groups, optional services, and provider payment rates. Other factors include the number of eligible individuals who enroll, utilization of covered services, and enrollment in other health insurance programs (including Medicare and private health insurance).

Figure 5 shows actual Medicaid expenditures from FY1997 to FY2017 and projected Medicaid expenditures from FY2018 through FY2026. These figures are broken down by state and federal expenditures. In FY2018, Medicaid spending on services and administrative activities in the 50 states, the District of Columbia, and the territories totaled $616 billion.[57] Medicaid expenditures are estimated to grow to $1,006 billion in FY2026.[58]

Historically, in a typical year, the average federal share of Medicaid expenditures was about 57%, which means the average state share was about 43%.

---

[57] CMS, CMS-64 Data, as of April 29, 2019.

[58] Christopher J. Truffer, Christian J. Wolfe, and Kathryn E. Rennie, *2017 Actuarial Report on the Financial Outlook for Medicaid*, Office of the Actuary, CMS, HHS, 2018.

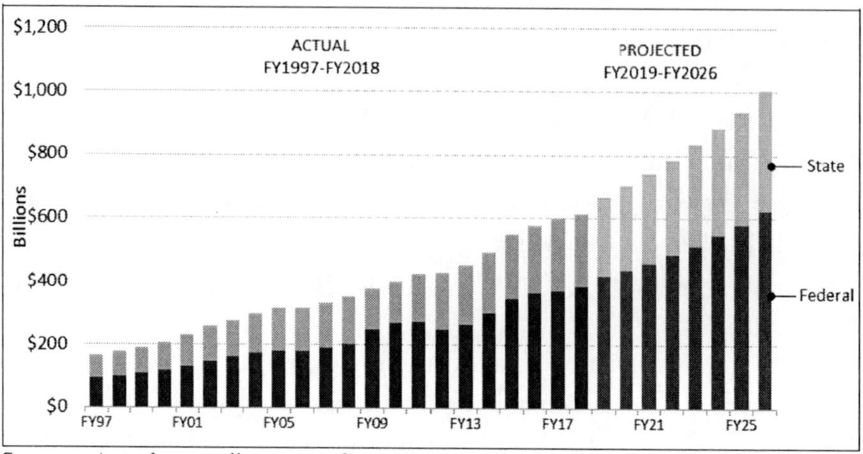

Sources: Actual expenditures are from Form CMS-64 Data as of April 29, 2019, and projected expenditures are from Christopher J. Truffer, Christian J. Wolfe, and Kathryn E. Rennie, 2017 Actuarial Report on the Financial Outlook for Medicaid, Office of the Actuary, CMS, HHS, 2018.

Note: The expenditures shown in this figure are total Medicaid expenditures, which include both administrative and benefit spending.

Figure 5. Federal and State Actual and Projected Medicaid Expenditures. (FY1997-FY2026)

However, the federal government's share of Medicaid expenditures increased with the implementation of the ACA Medicaid expansion, because the federal government is funding a vast majority of the cost of the expansion through the enhanced federal matching rates.[59] In FY2018, the average federal share of Medicaid is estimated to have been 62%, and it is expected to remain at that level through FY2026.[60]

With the implementation of the ACA Medicaid expansion in 2014, Medicaid expenditures increased 8.4% in FY2014 and 11.6% in FY2015.[61] But since then, Medicaid expenditure growth has slowed; some reasons for

---

[59] For more information about the enhanced federal matching rates for the ACA Medicaid expansion, see CRS In Focus IF10399, *Overview of the ACA Medicaid Expansion*.

[60] Christopher J. Truffer, Christian J. Wolfe, and Kathryn E. Rennie, *2017 Actuarial Report on the Financial Outlook for Medicaid*, Office of the Actuary, CMS, HHS, 2018.

[61] Christopher J. Truffer, Christian J. Wolfe, and Kathryn E. Rennie, *2016 Actuarial Report on the Financial Outlook for Medicaid*, Office of the Actuary, CMS, HHS, 2017; Christopher J. Truffer, Christian J. Wolfe, and Kathryn E. Rennie, *2015 Actuarial Report on the Financial Outlook for Medicaid*, Office of the Actuary, CMS, HHS, 2016.

this include slowing enrollment growth and managed care payment recoveries.[62] However, the rate of growth for Medicaid expenditures is expected to increase starting in 2019 due in part to additional states implementing the ACA Medicaid expansion and price factors.[63] This growth is expected to be somewhat offset by the reductions to Medicaid DSH allotments.[64]

MEDICAID PROGRAM WAIVERS

The Social Security Act authorizes several waiver and demonstration authorities to provide states with the flexibility to operate their Medicaid programs. Waiver authorities permit states to disregard certain requirements and operate their programs outside of Medicaid rules. Each waiver authority has a distinct purpose and specific requirements. Under the various waiver authorities, states may try new or different approaches to the delivery of health care services or adapt their programs to the special needs of particular geographic areas or groups of Medicaid enrollees. The primary Medicaid waiver authorities include the following:

- *Section 1115 Research and Demonstration Projects*—SSA Section 1115 authorizes the HHS Secretary to waive Medicaid requirements contained in SSA Section 1902 (including but not limited to rules regarding *freedom of choice* of provider, *comparability* of services, and *statewideness*) and/or provide expenditure authority for expenditures that do not otherwise qualify for federal financial participation under SSA Section 1903 (referred to as *costs not otherwise matchable*) in order to permit

---

[62] Anne B. Martin, Micah Hartman, and Benjamin Washington, et al., "National Health Care Spending in 2017: Growth Slows to Post-Great Recession Rates; Share of GDP Stabilizes," *Health Affairs*, vol. 38, no. 1 (January 2019).

[63] Andrea M. Sisko, Sean P. Keehan, and John A. Poisal, et al., "National Health Expenditure Projections, 2018-27: Economic and Demographic Trends Drive Spending and Enrollment Growth," *Health Affairs*, vol. 38, no. 3 (March 2019).

[64] Ibid. For more information about Medicaid DSH reductions, see CRS In Focus IF10422, *Medicaid Disproportionate Share Hospital (DSH) Reductions*.

states to conduct experimental, pilot, or demonstration projects that, in the judgment of the Secretary of HHS, are likely to assist in promoting the objectives of the Medicaid program. States use this waiver authority in a variety of ways, for example, to change eligibility criteria to offer coverage to new groups of people; to condition Medicaid eligibility on an enrollee's ability to meet work or other community engagement requirements; to provide services that are not otherwise covered, to offer different service packages or a combination of services in different parts of the state (e.g., coverage of nonelderly adults who are patients in institutions for mental disease);[65] to cap program enrollment, and to implement innovative service delivery systems.

- *Section 1915(b) Managed Care/Freedom of Choice Waivers*—SSA Section 1915(b) authorizes the HHS Secretary to waive the *freedom of choice* of provider requirement to establish mandatory managed care programs or otherwise limit enrollees' choice of providers.[66]
- *Section 1915(c) Home and Community-Based Services Waivers*—SSA Section 1915(c) authorizes the HHS Secretary to waive requirements regarding *comparability* of services and *statewideness* in covering a broad range of HCBS (including services not available under the Medicaid state plan) for certain persons with LTSS needs. States also may waive certain income and resource rules applicable to persons in the community, which means that a spouse's or parent's income and, to some extent, resources are not considered available to the applicant for the purposes of determining Medicaid financial eligibility. States may use Section

---

[65] For information about the institutions for mental disease exclusion, see CRS In Focus IF10222, *Medicaid's Institutions for Mental Disease (IMD) Exclusion*.

[66] There are four types of authorities under §1915(b) that states may request: (b)(1) allows states to require Medicaid beneficiaries to enroll in managed care; (b)(2) allows states to designate a "central broker" to assist Medicaid beneficiaries in choosing among competing health care plans; (b)(3) allows states to use cost savings made possible through the recipients' use of more cost-effective medical care to provide additional services; and (b)(4) allows states to limit the beneficiaries' choice of providers (except in emergency situations, for recipients residing in a long term care facility, and with respect to family planning services).

1915(c) concurrently with other waiver authorities. For example, states may combine Sections 1915(b) and 1915(c) authorities to offer mandatory managed care for HCBS.

Table 2. Key Characteristics of the Primary Medicaid Waiver Authorities Compared to State Plan Requirements

Key Characteristic	§1115 Research and Demonstration Waivers	§1915(b) Managed Care/Freedom of Choice Waivers	§1915(c) Home and Community-Based Services (HCBS) Waivers	Medicaid State Plan
Number of Waivers(as of May 2019)	60 waivers(in 44 states)[a]	78 waivers (in 38 states and DC)[b]	292 waivers (in 47 states and DC)[b]	N/A
Statewideness[c]	√	√	√	N/A
Comparability of Services[d]	√	√	√	N/A
Freedom of Choice of Provider[e]	√	√	—	N/A
Income and Resource Rules[f]	—	—	√	N/A
Federal Matching Funds for Costs Not Otherwise Matchable	√	√	√	N/A
Evaluations required	√	√	√	N/A
Duration	5 year initial, generally renewed for up to 3-year intervals (or up to 10 years for noncomplex waivers)	2 year initial, renewed for up to 2-year intervals	3 year initial, renewed for up to 5-year intervals	Once approved duration indefinite
Financing	Budget neutral over the life of the program	Must meet costeffectiveness test	Must meet costneutrality test	Open-ended mandatory entitlement
Enrollment caps and waiting lists permitted	√	—	√	

Source: Prepared by CRS based on program rules and regulations.

[a]This waiver count identifies operational Section 1115 demonstration programs as posted on the Centers for Medicare & Medicaid (CMS) website, as of May 2019. Operational waivers are defined as Section 1115 waivers that have been granted CMS approval (and agreed upon by the

state) for a current effective period as specified in the waiver Special Terms and Conditions (STCs), or as otherwise specified through a CMS waiver approval letter (e.g., a CMS approval letter that grants a temporary extension for all [or part] of the underlying demonstration waiver). This count may include waivers that are pending implementation as long as there is official documentation to show that the state has accepted the waiver conditions as outlined in the STCs and related documents (extension letters, amendment letters, etc.).

[b]The waiver counts for Section 1915(b) and (c) waiver programs are the number of waivers listed as "active" on the CMS website as of May 2019.

[c]Waiving the statewideness requirement (as permitted under §1902[a][1] of the Social Security Act [SSA]) allows states to target waivers to particular areas of the state where the need is greatest or where certain types of providers are available, for example.

[d]Waiving comparability of services (SSA §1902[a][10][B]) allows states to target waiver services to particular groups of individuals or to target services on the basis of disease or condition.

[e]Waiving the freedom of choice requirement (SSA §1902[a][23]) allows states to implement managed care delivery systems or otherwise limit choice of provider.

[f]Waiving income and resource rules applicable to the community (SSA §1902[a][10][C][i][III])) means that a spouse's or parent's income and, to some extent, resources are not considered available to the applicant for the purposes of determining Medicaid financial eligibility.

[g]States may seek CMS approval to provide expenditure authority for expenditures that do not otherwise qualify for federal financial participation under SSA §1903.

[h]This waiver count provides the number of Section 1915(b) and (c) waiver programs listed as "active" on the CMS website.

States often operate multiple waiver programs with their state plans. Key characteristics of these primary Medicaid waiver authorities compared with state plan requirements are summarized in Table 2.

The statutory requirements that may be waived under each type of waiver are different, but all types of waivers are time limited and approvals are subject to reporting and evaluation requirements. In addition, all types of waivers must comply with various financing requirements (e.g., budget neutrality, [67] cost-effectiveness,[68] or cost-neutrality[69]).

---

[67] *Budget neutrality* means the estimated spending under the waiver cannot exceed the estimated cost of the state's Medicaid program without the waiver.

[68] *Cost-effectiveness* means the cost of payments under managed care cannot exceed the cost of fee-for-service absent the waiver.

[69] Under the cost-neutrality test, expenditures under the waiver may not exceed the cost of institutional care that would have been provided to waiver recipients absent the waiver.

PROVIDER PAYMENTS

For the most part, states establish their own payment rates for Medicaid providers. Federal statute requires that these rates be consistent with efficiency, economy, and quality of care and sufficient to enlist enough providers so that covered benefits are available to Medicaid enrollees at least to the same extent they are available to the general population in the same geographic area.[70] This is known as the *equal access provision*.

Provider payment reductions are a tool for states to manage Medicaid program costs. As a result, states' provider rate changes are often a function of the economy. For instance, during the most recent recession, which ended in 2009, many states reduced Medicaid provider payment rates due to budget pressures. However, over the past couple years, more states have been enhancing rather than reducing provider rates overall due to improvements in state finances.[71] Low Medicaid provider payment rates in many states and their impact on provider participation have been perennial concerns for policymakers.[72]

In some cases, states make supplemental payments to Medicaid providers that are separate from, and in addition to, the payment rates for services rendered to Medicaid enrollees. Medicaid DSH payments are one type of supplemental payment, and federal statute requires that states make Medicaid DSH payments to hospitals treating large numbers of low-income patients.[73] States also are permitted to make non-DSH supplemental payments to providers, but these payments must adhere to

---

[70] SSA §1902(a)(30)(A).

[71] Kathleen Gifford, Eileen Ellis, Barbara Coulter Edwards, et al., *States Focus on Quality and Outcomes Amid Waiver Changes: Results from a 50-State Medicaid Budget Survey for State Fiscal Years 2018 and* 2019, Kaiser Commission on Medicaid and the Uninsured and the National Association of Medicaid Directors, October 2018.

[72] Sandra L. Decker, "In 2011 Nearly One-Third of Physicians Said They Would Not Accept New Medicaid Patients, But Rising Fees May Help," *Health Affairs*, vol. 31, no. 8 (August 2012), pp. 1673-1679.

[73] For more information about Medicaid DSH payments, see CRS Report R42865, *Medicaid Disproportionate Share Hospital Payments*.

upper payment limits (UPLs) for certain institutional providers.[74] The institutions subject to the UPL requirement are hospitals (separated into inpatient services and outpatient services), nursing facilities, intermediate care facilities for individuals with intellectual disabilities, and freestanding nonhospital clinics.[75]

PROGRAM INTEGRITY

Program integrity initiatives are designed to combat fraud, waste, and abuse in the Medicaid program. Some oversight efforts focus on preventing fraud and abuse through effective program management, while others focus on addressing problems after they occur through investigations, recoveries, and enforcement activities.

Multiple agencies at the federal and state levels are involved in program integrity. The federal agencies are CMS, the Office of the Inspector General for the Department of HHS, the Department of Justice, and the Government Accountability Office. The state agencies involved with program integrity activities include the state Medicaid agencies and the federally required Medicaid Fraud Control Units (MFCUs). Coordination of Medicaid program integrity activities can be a problem because there are so many agencies working on such initiatives and each state develops its own approach to program integrity.[76]

The federal government and states contribute equally to fund most Medicaid activities to combat waste, fraud, and abuse, although for some activities the federal government provides additional funds through enhanced FMAP rates. As mentioned earlier, all states receive the same FMAP rate for administrative expenditures, including most program

[74] Under the upper payment limit (UPL), federal Medicaid funding is not available for Medicaid payments that are more than Medicare would pay for the same or comparable services, and the UPL is an aggregate limit for each class of providers rather than a limit for individual providers.

[75] For more information about Medicaid supplemental payments, see CRS Report R45432, *Medicaid Supplemental Payments*.

[76] MACPAC, *Program Integrity*, at https://www.macpac.gov/subtopic/program-integrity/.

integrity activities, which generally is 50%. States receive higher FMAP rates for selected administrative activities, such as 90% for the startup of MFCUs and 75% for ongoing MFCU operation.

ADDITIONAL MEDICAID RESOURCES

This section provides links to a number of Medicaid resources grouped by background resources, laws, regulations, and other information.

Laws

Most federal Medicaid law is in SSA Title XIX (as amended): https://legcounsel.house.gov/Comps/Social%20Security%20Act-TITLE%20XIX(Grants%20to%20States%20for%20Medical%20Assistance%20Programs).pdf

SSA Title XIX is codified in the *U.S. Code* (42 U.S.C. §1396-1396w-5): http://uscode.house.gov/view.xhtml?path=/prelim@title42/chapter7/ subchapter19&edition= prelim

SSA Title XI has several general provisions relevant to Medicaid, including, for example, provisions on demonstration projects, the Center for Medicare & Medicaid Innovation, quality measures, and program integrity: https://legcounsel.house.gov/Comps/Social%20Security%20Act-TITLE%20XI(General%20Provisions,%20Peer%20Review,%20and%20Administrative%20Simp lification).pdf

SSA Title XI is codified in the *U.S. Code* (42 U.S.C. §§1301-1320e-3): http://uscode.house.gov/view.xhtml?path=/prelim@title42/chapter7/sub chapter11&edition= prelim

The entire SSA, as amended, is also available in a compilation from the House Office of Legislative Counsel

https://legcounsel.house.gov/Comps/SSA-merged.pdf

Regulations

Most federal Medicaid regulations are in Title 42 of the *Code of Federal Regulations* (42 C.F.R. §§430.0-456.725):

https://www.ecfr.gov/cgi-bin/text-idx?c=ecfr&tpl=/ecfrbrowse/Title42/42cfrv4_02.tpl

In addition to federal laws and regulations, CMS issues sub-regulatory program guidance through publications such as

- informational bulletins and letters to State Medicaid Directors https://www.medicaid.gov/federal-policy-Guidance/index.html
- the State Medicaid Manual https://www.cms.gov/Regulations-and-Guidance/Guidance/Manuals/PaperBased-Manuals-Items/CMS021927.html
- frequently asked questions https://www.medicaid.gov/faq/index.html

More Information

- Medicaid is administered at the federal level by CMS in HHS: https://www.cms.gov/
- CMS Office of the Actuary, "Medicaid: A Brief Summary," in *Brief Summaries of Medicare & Medicaid*: https://www.cms.gov/Research-Statistics-Data-and-Systems/Statistics-Trends-and-Reports/MedicareProgramRatesStats/SummaryMedicareMedicaid.html
- The federal Medicaid and CHIP Payment and Access Commission (MACPAC) publishes data and policy analysis and makes recommendations to Congress, the HHS Secretary, and states: https://www.macpac.gov/

- MACPAC, *Medicaid 101*: https://www.macpac.gov/Medicaid - 101/
- CMS, "Medicaid": https://www.medicaid.gov/medicaid/index.html
- MACPAC's "MACStats" compiles key national and state statistics from a variety of sources: https://www.macpac.gov/macstats/
- *CMS Fast Facts* has national statistics on beneficiaries, expenditures, and services: https://www.cms.gov/Research-Statistics-Data-and-Systems/Statistics-Trendsand-Reports/CMS-Fast-Facts/index.html

Each state operates its own Medicaid programs within federal guidelines.

- Links to information on each state's Medicaid program: https://www.medicaid.gov/state-overviews/index.html
- Links to each state's Medicaid website and contact information; scroll to "2. Through your state Medicaid agency": https://www.healthcare.gov/medicaid-chip/

In: Key Congressional Reports for June 2019 ISBN: 978-1-53616-665-1
Editor: Amada A. Byrd

Chapter 3

HEALTH CARE-RELATED EXPIRING PROVISIONS OF THE 116TH CONGRESS, FIRST SESSION*

Phoenix Voorhies, Kirsten J. Colello, Adrienne L. Fernandes, Bernadette Fernandez, Jim Hahn, Elayne J. Heisler, Paulette C. Morgan, Ryan J. Rosso, Amanda K. Sarata and Marco A. Villagrana

INTRODUCTION

This chapter describes selected health care-related provisions that are scheduled to expire during the first session of the116th Congress (i.e., during calendar year [CY] 2019).

---

* This is an edited, reformatted and augmented version of Congressional Research Service, Publication No. R45781, dated June 21, 2019.

For purposes of this chapter, *expiring provisions* are defined as portions of law that are time-limited and will lapse once a statutory deadline is reached absent further legislative action. The expiring provisions included in this chapter are those related to Medicare, Medicaid, State Children's Health Insurance Program (CHIP), and private health insurance programs and activities. The report also includes health care-related provisions that were enacted in the Patient Protection and Affordable Care Act (ACA; P.L. 111-148) or last extended under the Bipartisan Budget Act of 2018 (BBA 2018; P.L. 115-123). In addition, this chapter describes health care-related provisions within the same scope that expired during the 115th Congress (i.e., during CY2017 or CY2018).

This chapter generally focuses on two types of health care-related provisions within the scope discussed above. The first type of provision provides or controls mandatory spending, meaning that it provides temporary funding, temporary increases or decreases in funding (e.g., Medicare provider bonus payments), or temporary special protections that may result in changes in funding levels (e.g., Medicare funding provisions that establish a floor). The second type of provision defines the authority of government agencies or other entities to act, usually by authorizing a policy, project, or activity. Such provisions also may temporarily delay the implementation of a regulation, requirement, or deadline, or establish a moratorium on a particular activity. Expiring health care provisions that are predominantly associated with discretionary spending activities—such as discretionary authorizations of appropriations and authorities for discretionary user fees—are excluded from this chapter.

Certain types of provisions with expiration dates that otherwise would meet the criteria set forth above are excluded from this chapter. Some of these provisions are excluded because they are transitional or routine in nature or have been superseded by congressional action that otherwise modifies the intent of the expiring provision.

For example, statutorily required Medicare payment rate reductions and payment rate re-basings that are implemented over a specified time period are not considered to require legislative attention and are excluded.

The report provides tables listing the relevant provisions that are scheduled to expire in 2019 and that expired in 2018 or 2017. The report then describes each listed provision, including a legislative history. An appendix lists relevant demonstration projects and pilot programs that are scheduled to expire in 2019 or that expired in 2018 or 2017.

This chapter describes selected health care-related provisions that are scheduled to expire during the first session of the 116th Congress (i.e., during calendar year [CY] 2019). For purposes of this chapter, *expiring provisions* are defined as portions of law that are time-limited and will lapse once a statutory deadline is reached, absent further legislative action. The expiring provisions included in this chapter are those related to Medicare, Medicaid, State Children's Health Insurance Program (CHIP), and private health insurance programs and activities. The report also includes health care-related provisions that were enacted in the Patient Protection and Affordable Care Act (ACA; P.L. 111-148) or last extended under the Bipartisan Budget Act of 2018 (BBA 2018; P.L. 115-123). In addition, this chapter describes health care-related provisions within the same scope that expired during the 115th Congress (i.e., during CY2017 or CY2018).

This chapter generally focuses on two types of health care-related provisions within the scope discussed above. The first type of provision provides or controls mandatory spending, meaning that it provides temporary funding, temporary increases or decreases in funding (e.g., Medicare provider bonus payments), or temporary special protections that may result in changes in funding levels (e.g., Medicare funding provisions that establish a floor).

Mandatory spending is controlled by authorization acts; discretionary spending is controlled by appropriations acts.[1] The second type of provision defines the authority of government agencies or other entities to act, usually by authorizing a policy, project, or activity.[2] Such provisions also may temporarily delay the implementation of a regulation,

---

[1] For further information, see CRS Report R44582, *Overview of Funding Mechanisms in the Federal Budget Process, and Selected Examples*.

[2] For further information about these types of authorization provisions, see CRS Report R42098, *Authorization of Appropriations: Procedural and Legal Issues*.

requirement, or deadline, or establish a moratorium on a particular activity.[3] Expiring health care provisions that are predominantly associated with discretionary spending activities—such as discretionary authorizations of appropriations[4] and authorities for discretionary user fees—are excluded from this chapter.

Certain types of provisions with expiration dates that otherwise would meet the criteria set forth above are excluded from this chapter. Some of these provisions are excluded because they are transitional or routine in nature or have been superseded by congressional action that otherwise modifies the intent of the expiring provision. For example, statutorily required Medicare payment rate reductions and payment rate re-basings that are implemented over a specified time period are not considered to require legislative attention and are excluded.

The report is organized as follows: Table 1 lists the relevant provisions that are scheduled to expire in 2019. Table 2 lists the relevant provisions that expired during 2018 or 2017. The provisions in each table are organized by expiration date and applicable health care-related program.

The report then describes each listed provision, including a legislative history. The summaries are grouped by provisions that are scheduled to expire in 2019 followed by those that expired in 2018 or 2017.[5]

---

[3] Two private health insurance provisions included in this report do not meet the report criteria, but the provisons are expiring in 2019. Both provisions modify fees and taxes established by the Patient Protection and Affordable Care Act (ACA; P.L. 111-148, as amended) to help fund ACA activities, including those related to private health insurance.

[4] The Congressional Budget Office is required to compile this information each year under Section 202(e)(3) of the Congressional Budget Act. The most recent report, *Expired and Expiring Authorizations of Appropriations: Fiscal Year 2019* (March 14, 2019), which includes provisions set to expire on or before September 30, 2019, is available at https://www.cbo.gov/publication/55015.

[5] The 2019 expiring provisions are further organized by Social Security Act (SSA) and Public Health Service Act (PHSA) title and section. A third category includes provisions that are freestanding (i.e., new laws).

Table 1. Provisions Expiring in the 116th Congress, First Session

Expires After	Health Care Related Program	Provision[a]		Contact
9/30/2019	Medicaid	Protections for Recipients of Home and Community Based Services against Spouse Impoverishment	SSA §1924 42 U.S.C. §1296r-5	Kirsten Colello
9/30/2019	Medicaid	Additional Medicaid Funding for the Territories	SSA §1108 42 U.S.C. §1308	Alison Mitchel
9/30/2019	Medicare	Outreach and Assistance for Low-Income Programs	MIPPA §119 42 U.S.C. §1395b-3 note	Kirsten Colello
9/30/2019	Medicare	Temporary Extension of LTCH Site Neutral Payment Policy Transition Period	SSA §1886(m)(6)(B)(i) 42 U.S.C. §1395ww(m)(6)(B)(i)	Marco Villagrana
9/30/2019	Medicare	Temporary Exception for Certain Spinal Cord Conditions from Application of the Medicare LTCH Site Neutral Payment for Certain LTCHs	SSA §1886(m)(6)(F) 42 U.S.C. §1395ww(m)(6)(F)	Marco Villagrana
9/30/2019	Medicare	Funding for Implementation of Section 101 of MACRA	MACRA § 101(c)(3))	Jim Hahn
9/30/2019	Medicare	Priorities and Funding for Measure Development	SSA §1848(s) 42 U.S.C. §1395w-4(s)	Amanda Sarata
9/30/2019	Medicare	Contract with a Consensus Based Entity Regarding Performance Measurement	SSA §1890(d) 42 U.S.C. §1395aaa	Amanda Sarata
9/30/2019	Medicare	Quality Measure Selection	SSA §1890A 42 U.S.C. §1395aaa-1	Amanda Sarata
9/30/2019	Medicare	Patient-Centered Outcomes Research Trust Fund	IRC §9511 and §§4375-4377, SSA §1183); 26 U.S.C. §9511; 26 U.S.C.§§4375-4377; 42 U.S.C.§1320e-2	Amanda Sarata

Table 1. (Continued)

Expires After	Health Care Related Program	Provision[a]	Contact	
9/30/2019	Other	Family-to-Family Health Information Centers	SSA §501(c) 42 U.S.C. §701(c)(1)(A)(iii)	Elayne Heisler
9/30/2019	Other	Sexual Risk Avoidance Education Program	SSA §501 42 U.S.C. §710	Adrienne Fernandes Alcantara
9/30/2019	Other	Personal Responsibility Education Program	SSA §513 42 U.S.C. §713(f)	Adrienne Fernandes Alcantara
9/30/2019	Other	Pregnancy Assistance Fund	ACA §10212 42 U.S.C. §18201-18204	Adrienne Fernandes Alcantara
9/30/2019	Other	Teaching Health Centers	PHSA §340H 42 U.S.C. §256h	Elayne Heisler
9/30/2019	Other	Community Health Centers Fund	PHSA §330 42 U.S.C. §254b-2(b)(1)	Elayne Heisler
9/30/2019	Other	Special Diabetes Programs	PHSA §330B and §330C 42 U.S.C. §254c-2(b) and §254c-3(b)	Elayne Heisler
9/30/2019	Other	National Health Service Corps Appropriations	PHSA §338H 42 U.S.C. §254b-2(b)(2)	Elayne Heisler
9/30/2019	Other	Teaching Health Centers	PHSA §340H 42 U.S.C. §256h	Elayne Heisler
12/31/2019	Medicare	Floor on Work Geographic Practice Cost Indices	SSA §1848(e)(1) 42 U.S.C. §1395w-4(e)(1)(E)	Jim Hahn
12/31/2019	Medicare	Transitional Payment Rules for Certain Radiation Therapy Services	SSA §1848 42 U.S.C. 1395w-4(b)(11)	Jim Hahn
12/31/2019	Private Health Insurance	Health Coverage Tax Credit	IRC §35 26 U.S.C. §35	Bernadette Fernandez

Expires After	Health Care Related Program	Provision[a]	Contact	
12/31/2019	Private Health Insurance[b]	Annual Fee on Health Insurance Providers	ACA §9010	Ryan Rosso
12/31/2019	Private Health Insurance[b]	Excise Tax on Medical Device Manufacturers	26 U.S.C. §4191	Ryan Rosso

Source: Congressional Research Service (CRS).

Notes: ACA = Patient Protection and Affordable Care Act (P.L. 111-148. as amended), CY = Calendar Year, IRC = Internal Revenue Code, LTCH= Long-Term Care Hospital, MACRA = Medicare Access and CHIP Reauthorization Act of 2015, MIPPA = Medicare Improvements for Patients and Providers Act, PHSA = Public Health Service Act, SSA = Social Security Act, U.S.C. = *U.S. Code*.

[a]Citations in statute and the *United States Code* (U.S.C.) are provided where available.

[b]These two provisions did not meet the criteria for the report, but the provisions are expiring in 2019. Both provisions modify fees and taxes established by the Patient Protection and Affordable Care Act (ACA; P.L. 111-148, as amended) to help fund ACA activities, including those related to private health insurance.

Table 2. Provisions That Expired in the 115th Congress (CY2017 and CY2018)

Expired After	Health Care Related Program	Provision[a]		Contact
9/30/2017	Medicare	Delay in Applying the 25% Patient Threshold Payment Adjustment for Long-Term Care Hospitals	MMSEA §114(c) 42 U.S.C. §1395ww note	Marco Villagrana
9/30/2017	Medicare	Long-Term Care Hospital Moratoria	MMSEA §114(d) 42 U.S.C. §1395ww note	Marco Villagrana
12/31/2017	Medicare	Extension of Enforcement Instruction on Supervision Requirements for Outpatient Therapeutic Services in Critical Access and Small Rural Hospitals	P.L. 113-198	Jim Hahn

Table 2. (Continued)

Expires After	Health Care Related Program	Provision[a]	Contact	
9/30/2018	Medicare	Temporary Exception for Certain Severe Wound Discharges from Application of the Medicare Site Neutral Payment for Certain Long Term Care Hospitals	SSA §1886(m)(6)(E) and (G) 42 U.S.C. §1395ww(m)(6)(E) and (G)	Marco Villagrana
12/31/2018	Medicare	Exclusion of ASC Physicians from the Medicare Meaningful Use Payment Adjustment	SSA §1848(a)(7)(D) 42 U.S.C. §1395w–4(a)(7)(D)	Jim Hahn
12/31/2018	Medicare	Delay in Authority to Terminate Contracts for MA Plans Failing to Achieve Minimum Quality Ratings	SSA §1857 42 U.S.C. §1395w-27	Paulette Morgan

Source: Congressional Research Service.

Notes: ASC = Ambulatory Surgery Centers, CY = Calendar Year, MA = Medicare Advantage, MMSEA = Medicare, Medicaid, and SCHIP Extension Act of 2007, SSA = Social Security Act, U.S.C. = *U.S. Code*.

[a] Citations in statute and the *United States Code* (U.S.C.) are provided where available.

Appendix A lists demonstration projects and pilot programs that are scheduled to expire in 2019 or that expired in 2018 or 2017 and are related to Medicare, Medicaid, CHIP, and private health insurance programs and activities or other health care-related provisions that were enacted in the ACA or last extended under the BBA 2018. Appendix B lists all laws that created, modified, or extended the health care-related expiring provisions described in this chapter. Appendix C lists abbreviations used in the report.

CY2019 Expiring Provisions

Social Security Act (SSA) Title V: Sexual Risk Avoidance Education Program, Personal Responsibility Education Program, and Pregnancy Assistance Fund

Family-to-Family Health Information Centers (SSA §501(c); 42 U.S.C. §701(c)(1)(A)(iii))[6]

Background

The Family-to-Family Health Information Centers program funds family-staffed and family-run centers in the 50 states, the District of Columbia, the territories, and through a tribal organization. The Family-to-Family Health Information Centers provide information, education, technical assistance, and peer support to families of children (including youth) with special health care needs and health professionals who serve such families. They also assist in ensuring that families and health professionals are partners in decision-making at all levels of care and service delivery. This program is administered by the Health Resources and Services Administration (HRSA).

Relevant Legislation

- The Deficit Reduction Act of 2005 (DRA; P.L. 109-171), Section 6064, established the Family-to-Family Health Information Centers program in the 50 states and the District of Columbia and provided $3 million for FY2007, $4 million for FY2008, and $5 million for FY2009.
- ACA, Section 5507, provided $5 million for each of FY2009 through FY2012.
- The American Taxpayer Relief Act of 2012 (ATRA; P.L. 112-240), Section 624, provided $5 million for FY2013.

---

[6] Citations in statute and the *U.S. Code* (U.S.C.) are provided where available.

- The Pathway for SGR (Sustainable Growth Rate) Reform Act of 2013 (PSRA; P.L. 113-67, Division B), Section 1203, provided \$2.5 million for October 1, 2013, through March 31, 2014.
- The Protecting Access to Medicare Act of 2014 (PAMA; P.L. 113-93), Section 207, provided \$2.5 million for the remainder of FY2014 (from April 1, 2014, to September 30, 2014) and provided \$2.5 million for the first half of FY2015 (October 1, 2014, through March 31, 2015).
- The Medicare Access and CHIP Reauthorization Act of 2015 (MACRA; P.L. 114-10), Section 216, struck the partial funding provided in PAMA and provided full-year funding of \$5 million for FY2015. It also provided \$5 million for each of FY2016 and FY2017.
- BBA 2018, Section 50501, expanded the program to require that centers be developed in all of the territories and for at least one Indian tribe. It also provided \$6 million for each of FY2018 and FY2019.

Current Status

Appropriated funds to create or maintain Family-to-Family Health Information Centers have been enacted for FY2019, but under current law no new funding will be available for FY2020 or subsequent fiscal years.

Sexual Risk Avoidance Education Program (SSA §510; 42 U.S.C. §710)

Background

The Title V Sexual Risk Avoidance Education (SRAE) program, formerly known as the Abstinence Education Grants program, provides funding for education to adolescents aged 10 to 20 exclusively on abstaining from sexual activity outside of marriage.[7] Funding is provided

[7] A discretionary federal program has the same name, Sexual Risk Avoidance Education program. The programs are distinguished here by referring to the mandatory program as the

primarily via formula grants. The 50 states, District of Columbia, and the territories are eligible to apply for funds. Jurisdictions request Title V SRAE funds as part of their request for Maternal and Child Health Block Grant funds authorized in SSA Section 501. Funds are allocated to jurisdictions based on their relative shares of low-income children. Funding is also available for eligible entities (not defined in statute) in jurisdictions that do not apply for funding.

Relevant Legislation

- The Personal Responsibility and Work Opportunity Reconciliation Act of 1996 (PRWORA; P.L. 104-193), Section 912, established the Abstinence Education Grants program and provided $50 million for each of FY1998 through FY2002.
- The Welfare Reform Extension Act of 2003 (WREA 2003; P.L. 108-40), Section 6, provided $50 million for FY2003.
- P.L. 108-89, Section 101, provided funding through March 31, 2014 in the manner authorized for FY2002 (i.e., $50 million, but proportionally provided for the first two quarters of FY2004).
- The Welfare Reform Extension Act of 2004 (WREA 2004, P.L. 108-210), Section 2, provided funding through June 30, 2004 in the manner authorized for FY2002.
- P.L. 108-262, Section 2, provided funding through September 30, 2004 in the manner authorized for FY2002.
- P.L. 108-308, Section 2, provided funding through March 31, 2005 in the manner authorized for FY2004.
- The Welfare Reform Extension Act of 2005 (WREA 2005, P.L. 109-4), Section 2, provided funding through June 30, 2005 in the manner authorized for FY2004.
- P.L. 109-19, Section 2, provided funding through September 30, 2005 in the manner authorized for FY2004.

Title V Sexual Risk Avoidance Education program. For further information about both programs, see CRS Report R45183, *Teen Pregnancy: Federal Prevention Programs*.

- P.L. 109-91, Section 102, provided funding through December 31, 2005 in the manner authorized for FY2005.

The Tax Relief and Health Care Act of 2006 (TRHCA; P.L. 109-432), Section 401, provided funding through June 30, 2007 in the manner authorized for FY2006.

- P.L. 110-48, Section 1, provided funding through September 30, 2007 in the manner authorized for FY2006.
- P.L. 110-90, Section 2, provided funding through December 31, 2007 in the manner authorized for FY2007.
- The Medicare, Medicaid, and SCHIP Extension Act of 2007 (MMSEA; P.L. 110-173), Section 202, provided funding through June 30, 2008 in the manner authorized for FY2007.
- The Medicare Improvements for Patients and Providers Act of 2008 (MIPPA, P.L. 110-275), Section 201, provided funding through June 30, 2009 in the manner authorized for FY2007.
- ACA, Section 2954, provided $50 million for each of FY2010 through FY2014.
- PAMA, Section 205, provided $50 million for FY2015.
- MACRA, Section 214, provided $75 million for each of FY2016 and FY2017.
- BBA 2018, Section 50502, renamed the program and provided $75 million for each of FY2018 and FY2019.

Current Status

Appropriated funds for the Title V SRAE program have been enacted for FY2019, but under current law no new funding will be available for FY2020 or subsequent fiscal years.

Personal Responsibility Education Program (SSA §513; 42 U.S.C. §713(f))

Background

The Personal Responsibility Education Program (PREP) takes a broad approach to teen pregnancy prevention that targets adolescents aged 10 to 20 and pregnant and parenting youth under the age of 21.[8] Education services can address abstinence and/or contraceptives to prevent pregnancy and sexually transmitted infections. PREP includes four types of grants: (1) State PREP grants, (2) Competitive PREP grants, (3) Tribal PREP, and (4) PREP–Innovative Strategies (PREIS). A majority of PREP funding is allocated to states and territories via the State PREP grant. The 50 states, District of Columbia, and the territories are eligible for funding. Funds are allocated by formula based on the proportion of youth aged 10 to 20 in each jurisdiction relative to other jurisdictions.

Relevant Legislation

- ACA, Section 2953, established PREP and provided $75 million annually from FY2010 through FY2014.
- PAMA, Section 206, provided $75 million for FY2015.
- MACRA, Section 215, provided $75 million for each of FY2016 and FY2017.
- BBA 2018, Section 50503, provided $75 million for each of FY2018 and FY2019.

Current Status

Appropriated funds for PREP have been enacted for FY2019, but under current law no new funding will be available for FY2020 or subsequent fiscal years.

---

[8] For further information about PREP, see CRS Report R45183, *Teen Pregnancy: Federal Prevention Programs.*

Pregnancy Assistance Fund (ACA §10212; 42 U.S.C. §18201-18204)

The Pregnancy Assistance Fund (PAF) program seeks to improve the educational, health, and social outcomes of vulnerable individuals who are expectant or new parents and their children. PAF funding is awarded competitively to the 50 states, District of Columbia, the territories, and tribal entities that apply successfully. The grantees may use the funds for providing subgrants to community service providers and selected other entities that provide services during the prenatal and postnatal periods. Grantees may also provide, in partnership with the state attorney general's office, certain legal and other services for women who experience domestic violence, sexual assault, or stalking while they are pregnant or parenting an infant. Further, grant funds can be used to support public awareness efforts about PAF services for the expectant and parenting population.

Relevant Legislation

- ACA, Section 10212, established the PAF program and provided $25 million for each of FY2010 through FY2019.

Current Status

Appropriated funds for the PAF program funds have been enacted for FY2019, but under current law no new funding will be available for FY2020 or subsequent fiscal years.

SSA Title VXIII: Medicare

Temporary Extension of Long-Term Care Hospital (LTCH) Site Neutral Payment Policy Transition Period (SSA §1886(m)(6)(B)(i); 42 U.S.C. §1395ww(m)(6)(B)(i))

Background

Medicare pays LTCHs for certain inpatient hospital care under the LTCH prospective payment system (LTCH PPS), which is typically higher than payments for inpatient hospital care under the inpatient prospective payment system (IPPS). PSRA amended the law so that the LTCH PPS payment is no longer available for all LTCH discharges but instead is available only for those LTCH discharges that met specific clinical criteria. Specifically, LTCHs are paid under the LTCH PPS if a Medicare beneficiary either (1) had a prior three-day intensive-care-unit stay at a hospital paid under the IPPS immediately preceding the LTCH stay or (2) is assigned to an LTCH PPS case-mix group that is based on the receipt of ventilator services for at least 96 hours and had a prior hospital stay at a hospital paid under the IPPS immediately preceding the LTCH stay. Discharges involving patients who have a principal diagnosis relating to a psychiatric diagnosis or rehabilitation do not qualify for the LTCH PPS rate. (Subsequent legislation provided for other criteria to temporarily receive payment under the LTCH PPS. See sections "Temporary Exception for Certain Spinal Cord Conditions from Application of the Medicare LTCH Site Neutral Payment for Certain LTCHs (SSA §1886(m)(6)(F); 42 U.S.C. §1395ww(m)(6)(F))" and "Temporary Exception for Certain Severe Wound Discharges from Application of the Medicare Site Neutral Payment for Certain Long Term Care Hospitals (SSA §1886(m)(6)(E) and (G); 42 U.S.C. §1395ww(m)(6)(E) and (G))" below.)

For LTCH discharges that did not qualify for the LTCH PPS based on these clinical criteria, a "site neutral payment rate" similar to the PPS for inpatient acute care hospitals (IPPS) was to be phased-in. The site neutral rate is defined as the lower of an "IPPS-comparable" per diem amount, as defined in regulations, or the estimated cost of the services involved.

Relevant Legislation

- PSRA, Section 1206(a), established patient criteria for payment under the LTCH PPS and a site-neutral payment rate for LTCH patients who do not meet these criteria. During a phase-in period for discharges in cost-reporting periods beginning in FY2016 and FY2017, LTCHs received a blended payment amount based on 50% of what the LTCH would have been reimbursed under the

LTCH PPS rate and 50% of the site neutral payment rate. For cost-reporting periods beginning in FY2018 and subsequent years, the LTCH was to receive the site neutral payment rate.

- BBA 2018, Section 51005, extended the transition period to site neutral Medicare payments for LTCH patients who do not meet the patient criteria for an additional two years, to include discharges in cost-reporting periods beginning during FY2018 and FY2019. During this period, LTCHs continue to receive the 50/50 blended payment for discharges that do not meet certain LTCH PPS criteria.

Current Status

The extended transition period to site neutral payments during which LTCHs receive a blended payment for discharges that do not meet the patient criteria expires for discharges occurring in cost-reporting periods beginning during FY2020 and subsequent years.

Temporary Exception for Certain Spinal Cord Conditions from Application of the Medicare LTCH Site Neutral Payment for Certain LTCHs (SSA §1886(m)(6)(F); 42 U.S.C. §1395ww(m)(6)(F))

Background

Medicare pays LTCHs for inpatient hospital care under the LTCH PPS, which is typically higher than payments for inpatient hospital care under the IPPS. Effective for cost-reporting periods beginning in FY2016, LTCHS are paid the LTCH PPS rate for patients that meet one of the following two criteria: (1) had a prior three-day intensive-care-unit stay at a hospital paid under the IPPS immediately preceding the LTCH stay or (2) is assigned to an LTCH PPS case-mix group that is based on the receipt of ventilator services for at least 96 hours and had a prior hospital stay at a hospital paid under the IPPS immediately preceding the LTCH stay. Discharges involving patients who have a principal diagnosis relating to a psychiatric diagnosis or rehabilitation do not qualify for the LTCH PPS rate. For LTCH discharges that did not qualify for the LTCH PPS based on these criteria, a site neutral payment rate is being phased-in for cost-reporting periods beginning FY2016 through FY2019. Subsequent legislation provided for other criteria to temporarily receive payment under the LTCH PPS. See section "Temporary Extension of Long-Term Care Hospital (LTCH) Site Neutral Payment Policy Transition Period (SSA §1886(m)(6)(B)(i); 42 U.S.C. §1395ww(m)(6)(B)(i))" for details related to site neutral payment.

Relevant Legislation

- The 21st Century Cures Act (Cures Act; P.L. 114-255), Division C, Section 15009 established an additional temporary criterion for payment under the LTCH PPS related to certain spinal cord conditions for discharges occurring in cost-reporting periods FY2018 and FY2019. Specifically, the LTCH PPS rate would apply to an LTCH discharge if all of the following are met: (1) the LTCH was a not-for-profit on June 1, 2014; (2) at least 50% of the LTCH's CY2013 LTCH PPS-paid discharges were classified under LTCH diagnosis related groups (DRGs) associated with catastrophic spinal cord injuries, acquired brain injury, or other paralyzing neuromuscular conditions; and (3) the LTCH during FY2014 discharged patients (including Medicare beneficiaries and others) who had been admitted from at least 20 of the 50 states, as determined by the Secretary of Health and Human Services (HHS) based on a patient's state of residency.

Current Status

The authority for the temporary criterion related to certain spinal cord conditions to receive payment under the LTCH PPS expires for discharges occurring in cost reporting periods beginning during FY2020 and subsequent years.

Funding for Implementation of Section 101 of MACRA (MACRA Section 101(c)(3))

Background

Section 101 of MACRA made fundamental changes to the way Medicare payments to physicians are determined and how they are updated.[9] To implement the payment modifications in Section 101 of MACRA, the law authorized the transfer of $80 million from the Supplementary Medical Insurance (SMI) Trust Fund for each fiscal year beginning with FY2015 and ending with FY2019. The amounts transferred are to be available until expended.

Relevant Legislation

- MACRA, Section 101, provided for the transfer of $80 million, for each of FY2015 through FY2019, from the Medicare SMI Trust Fund.

Current Status

Appropriated funds to support the activities under this subsection have not been enacted for FY2020 or subsequent fiscal years.

Priorities and Funding for Measure Development (SSA §1848(s); 42 U.S.C. §1395w-4(s))

Background

SSA Section 1848(s) required the HHS Secretary to develop a plan for the development of quality measures for use in the Merit-based Incentive Payment System program, which is to be updated as needed. The subsection also requires the Secretary to enter into contracts or other arrangements to develop, improve, update, or expand quality measures, in accordance with the plan. In entering into contracts, the Secretary must

---

[9] For more information on Section 101 of MACRA, see CRS Report R43962, *The Medicare Access and CHIP Reauthorization Act of 2015 (MACRA; P.L. 114-10).*

give priority to developing measures of outcomes, patient experience of care, and care coordination, among other things. The HHS Secretary, through the Center for Medicare & Medicaid Services (CMS), annually reports on the progress made in developing quality measures under this subsection.

Relevant Legislation

- MACRA, Section 102, provided for the transfer of $15 million, for each of FY2015 through FY2019, from the Medicare SMI Trust Fund.

Current Status

Appropriated funds to support the activities under this subsection have not been enacted for FY2020 or subsequent fiscal years. However, funds appropriated prior to FY2020 are available for obligation through the end of FY2022.

Contract with a Consensus-Based Entity Regarding Performance Measurement (SSA §1890(d); 42 U.S.C. §1395aaa)

Background

Under SSA Section 1890, the HHS Secretary is required to have a contract with a consensus-based entity (e.g., National Quality Forum, or NQF) to carry out specified duties related to performance improvement and measurement. These duties include, among others, priority setting, measure endorsement, measure maintenance, and annual reporting to Congress.

Relevant Legislation

- MIPPA, Section 183, transferred, from the Medicare hospital insurance (HI) and SMI Trust Funds, a total of $10 million for each of FY2009 through FY2012 to carry out the activities under SSA Section 1890.

- ATRA, Section 609(a), provides $10 million for FY2013 and modified the duties of the consensus-based entity.
- PSRA, Section 1109, required that transferred funding remain available until expended.
- PAMA, Section 109, transferred $5 million for the remainder of FY2014 (from April 1, 2014, to September 30, 2014) and $15 million for the first six months of FY2015 (from October 1, 2014, to March 31, 2015) to carry out both SSA Section 1890 and SSA Section 1890A(a)-(d); funds were required to remain available until expended.
- MACRA, Section 207, transferred $30 million for each of FY2015 through FY2017 to carry out both SSA Section 1890 and SSA Section 1890A(a)-(d). The funding provided under MACRA for FY2015 effectively replaced the funding provided under PAMA for that year; therefore, the total funding for FY2015 was $30 million. Funds were required to remain available until expended.
- BBA 2018, Section 50206, transferred $7.5 million from the Medicare HI and SMI Trust Funds for each of FY2018 and FY2019 to carry out both Section 1890 and SSA Section 1890A(a)-(d). The section also added new HHS reporting requirements and modified existing NQF reporting requirements to specify use of funding, among other things. Amounts transferred for each of FY2018 and FY2019 are in addition to any unobligated balances that remained from prior years' transfers.

Current Status

Appropriated funds to support the contract with the consensus-based entity from SSA Section 1890 have not been enacted for FY2020 or subsequent fiscal years. However, funds appropriated prior to FY2020 are available for obligation until expended.

Quality Measure Selection (SSA §1890A; 42 U.S.C. §1395aaa-1)

Background

SSA Section 1890A requires the HHS Secretary to establish a pre-rulemaking process to select quality measures for use in the Medicare program. As part of this process, the Secretary makes available to the public measures under consideration for use in Medicare quality programs and broadly disseminates the quality measures that are selected to be used, while the consensus-based entity with a contract (NQF) gathers multi-stakeholder input and annually transmits that input to the Secretary. NQF fulfills this requirement through its Measure Applications Partnership (MAP), an entity that convenes multi-stakeholder groups to provide input into the selection of quality measures for use in Medicare and other federal programs. MAP publishes annual reports with recommendations for selection of quality measures in February of each year, with the first report published in February 2012.

Relevant Legislation

- ACA, Section 3014(c), transferred a total of $20 million from the Medicare HI and SMI Trust Funds for each of FY2010 through FY2014 to carry out SSA Section 1890A(a)-(d) (and the amendments made to SSA Section 1890(b) by ACA Section 3014(a)).
- PAMA, Section 109, transferred $5 million for the remainder of FY2014 (from April 1, 2014, to September 30, 2014) and $15 million for the first six months of FY2015 (from October 1, 2014, to March 31, 2015) to carry out both SSA Section 1890 and SSA Section 1890A(a)-(d); funds were required to remain available until expended.
- MACRA, Section 207, transferred $30 million for each of FY2015 through FY2017 to carry out both SSA Section 1890 and SSA Section 1890A(a)-(d). The funding provided under MACRA for

FY2015 replaced the funding provided under PAMA for that year; therefore, the total funding for FY2015 was $30 million.

- BBA 2018, Section 50206, transferred $7.5 million for each of FY2018 and FY2019 to carry out both Section 1890 and SSA Section 1890A(a)-(d). The section also added new HHS reporting requirements and modified existing NQF reporting requirements to specify use of funding, among other things. Amounts transferred for each of FY2018 and FY2019 are in addition to any unobligated balances that remained from prior years' transfers.

Current Status

Appropriated funds to carry out the measure selection activities from SSA Section 1890A(a)-(d) have not been enacted for FY2020 or subsequent fiscal years. However, funds appropriated prior to FY2020 are available for obligation until expended.

Floor on Work Geographic Practice Cost Indices (SSA §1848(e)(1); 42 U.S.C. §1395w-4(e)(1)(E))

Background

Payments under the Medicare physician fee schedule (MPFS) are adjusted geographically for three factors to reflect differences in the cost of resources needed to produce physician services: physician work, practice expense, and medical malpractice insurance. The geographic adjustments are indices—known as Geographic Practice Cost Indices (GPCIs)—that reflect how each area compares to the national average in a "market basket" of goods. A value of 1.00 represents the average across all areas. These indices are used in the calculation of the payment rate under the MPFS. Several laws have established a minimum value of 1.00 (floor) for the physician work GPCI for localities where the work GPCI was less than 1.00.

Relevant Legislation

- Medicare Prescription Drug, Improvement, and Modernization Act of 2003 (MMA, P.L. 108-173), Section 412, provided for an increase in the work geographic index to 1.0 (floor) for any locality for which the work geographic index was less than 1.0 for services furnished from January 1, 2004, through December 31, 2006.
- TRHCA, Section 102, extended the floor through December 31, 2007.
- MMSEA, Section 103, extended the floor through June 30, 2008.
- MIPPA, Section 134, extended the floor through December 31, 2009. In addition, beginning January 1, 2009, MIPAA set the work geographic index for Alaska to 1.5 if the index otherwise would be less than 1.5; no expiration was set for this modification.
- ACA, Section 3102, extended the floor through December 31, 2010.
- Medicare and Medicaid Extenders Act of 2010 (MMEA, P.L. 111-309), Section 103, extended the floor through December 31, 2011.
- Temporary Payroll Tax Cut Continuation Act of 2011 (TPTCCA, P.L. 112- 78), Section 303, extended the floor through February 29, 2012.
- Middle Class Tax Relief and Job Creation Act of 2012 (MCTRJCA, P.L. 112- 96), Section 3004, extended the floor through December 31, 2012, and required the Medicare Payment Advisory Commission (MedPAC) to report on whether any work geographic adjustment to the MPFS is appropriate, what that level of adjustment should be (if appropriate), and where the adjustment should be applied. The report also was required to assess the impact of such an adjustment, including how it would affect access to care.
- ATRA, Section 602, extended the floor through December 31, 2013.

- PAMA, Section 102, extended the floor through March 31, 2015.
- MACRA, Section 201, extended the floor through December 31, 2017.
- BBA 2018, Section 50201, extended the floor through December 31, 2019.

Current Status

The authority for the MPFS GPCI floor will expire after December 31, 2019.

Transitional Payment Rules for Certain Radiation Therapy Services (SSA §1848(b)(11); 42 U.S.C. §1395w-4(b)(11))

Background

Currently, Medicare payments for services of physicians and certain non-physician practitioners, including radiation therapy services, are made on the basis of a fee schedule.

To set payment rates under the MPFS, relative values units (RVUs) are assigned to each of more than 7,000 service codes that reflect physician work (i.e., the time, skill, and intensity it takes to provide the service), practice expenses, and malpractice costs. The relative value for a service compares the relative work and other inputs involved in performing one service with the inputs involved in providing other physicians' services. The relative values are adjusted for geographic variation in input costs. The adjusted relative values are then converted into a dollar payment amount by a conversion factor.

CMS, which is responsible for maintaining and updating the fee schedule, continually modifies and refines the methodology for estimating RVUs. CMS is required to review the RVUs no less than every five years; the ACA added the requirement that the HHS Secretary periodically identify physician services as being potentially misvalued, and make appropriate adjustments to the relative values of such services under the Medicare physician fee schedule.

In determining adjustments to RVUs used as the basis for calculating Medicare physician reimbursement under the fee schedule, the HHS Secretary has authority, under previously existing law and as augmented by the ACA, to adjust the number of RVUs for any service code to take into account changes in medical practice, coding changes, new data on relative value components, or the addition of new procedures.

Under the potentially misvalued codes authority, certain radiation therapy codes were identified as being potentially misvalued in 2015. However, because of concerns that the existing code set did not accurately reflect the radiation therapy treatments identified, CMS created several new codes during the transition toward an episodic alternative payment model.

Relevant Legislation

- Patient Access and Medicare Protection Act (PAMPA; P.L. 114-115) required CMS to apply the same code definitions, work RVUs, and direct inputs for the practice expense RVUs in CY2017 and CY2018 as applied in 2016 for these transition codes, effectively keeping the payments for these services unchanged, subject to the annual update factor. PAMPA exempted these radiation therapy and related imaging services from being considered as potentially misvalued services under CMS's misvalued codes initiative for CY2017 and CY2018. PAMPA also instructed the HHS Secretary to report to Congress on the development of an episodic alternative payment model under the Medicare program for radiation therapy services furnished in non-facility settings.
- BBA 2018 Section 51009, extended the restrictions through CY2019.

Current Status

The payment restrictions expire after December 31, 2019.

Other Medicare Provisions

Outreach and Assistance for Low-Income Programs (MIPPA §119; 42 U.S.C. §1395b-3 note)

Background

The Administration for Community Living (ACL) administers federal grant programs that fund outreach and assistance to older adults, individuals with disabilities, and their caregivers in accessing various health and social services. Funding for these programs is provided through discretionary budget authority in annual appropriations to the following entities:

- State Health Insurance Assistance Programs (SHIPs): programs that provide outreach, counseling, and information assistance to Medicare beneficiaries and their families and caregivers on Medicare and other health insurance issues.
- Area Agencies on Aging (AAA): state-designated public or private nonprofit agencies that address the needs and concerns of older adults at the regional or local levels. AAAs plan, develop, coordinate, and deliver a wide range of home and community-based services. Most AAAs are direct providers of information and referral assistance programs.
- Aging and Disability Resource Centers (ADRCs): programs in local communities that assist older adults, individuals with disabilities, and caregivers in accessing the full range of long-term services and supports options, including available public programs and private payment options.

The National Center for Benefits and Outreach Enrollment assists organizations to enroll older adults and individuals with disabilities into benefit programs that they may be eligible for, such as Medicare, Medicaid, the Supplemental Security Income (SSI) program, and the Supplemental Nutrition Assistance Program (SNAP), among others.

In addition to discretionary funding for these programs, beginning in FY2009, MIPPA provided funding for specific outreach and assistance activities to Medicare beneficiaries. This mandatory funding was extended multiple times, most recently in BBA 2018 through FY2019, and provided for outreach and assistance to low-income Medicare beneficiaries including those who may be eligible for the Low-Income Subsidy program, Medicare Savings Program (MSP), and the Medicare Part D Prescription Drug Program. The HHS Secretary is required to transfer specified amounts for MIPPA program activities from the Medicare Trust Funds.[10]

BBA 2018 also requires ACL[11] to electronically post on its website by April 1, 2019, and biennially thereafter, the following information with respect to SHIP state grants: (1) the amount of federal funding provided to each state and the amount of federal funding provided by each state to each entity and (2) other program information, as specified by the HHS Secretary. Publicly reported information must be presented by state as well as by entity receiving funds from the state.

Relevant Legislation

- MIPPA, Section 119, authorized and provided a total of $25 million for FY2009 to fund low-income Medicare beneficiary outreach and education activities through SHIPs, AAAs, ADRCs, and coordination efforts to inform older Americans about benefits available under federal and state programs.
- ACA, Section 3306, extended authority for these programs and provided a total of $45 million for FY2010 through FY2012 in the following amounts: SHIPs, $15 million; AAAs, $15 million; ADRCs, $10 million; and the contract with the National Center for Benefits and Outreach Enrollment, $5 million.

---

[10] Medicare has two trust funds: the Hospital Insurance (HI) Trust Fund and the Supplementary Medical Insurance (SMI) Trust Fund. The HI Trust Fund finances Medicare Part A services, including hospital, home health, skilled nursing facility, and hospice care. The SMI Trust Fund finances Medicare Parts B and D, including physician and outpatient hospital services and outpatient prescription drugs.

[11] Section 50207 of BBA 2018 refers to the "Agency for Community Living."

- ATRA, Section 610, extended authority for these programs through FY2013 and provided a total of $25 million in the following amounts: SHIPs, $7.5 million; AAAs, $7.5 million; ADRCs, $5 million; and the contract with the National Center for Benefits and Outreach Enrollment, $5 million.
- PSRA, Section 1110, extended authority for these programs through the second quarter of FY2014 and provided funds at FY2013 levels ($25 million) for the first two quarters of FY2014 (through March 31, 2014).
- PAMA, Section 110, extended authority for these programs through the second quarter of FY2015 (through March 31, 2015). For FY2014, PAMA provided a total of $25 million at the following FY2013 funding levels: SHIPs, $7.5 million; AAAs, $7.5 million; ADRCs, $5.0 million; and the contract with the National Center for Benefits and Outreach Enrollment, $5.0 million. In addition, PAMA provided funds at FY2014 levels for the first two quarters of FY2015 (through March 31, 2015).
- MACRA, Section 208, extended authority for these programs through September 30, 2017. For FY2015, MACRA provided funding at the previous year's level of $25 million in the following amounts: SHIPs, $7.5 million; AAAs, $7.5 million; ADRCs, $5 million; and the contract with the National Center for Benefits and Outreach Enrollment, $5 million. For FY2016 and FY2017, MACRA provided $37.5 million annually, a $12.5 million per year increase from FY2015 funding levels, in the following amounts: SHIPs, $13 million; AAAs, $7.5 million; ADRCs, $5 million; and the contract with the National Center for Benefits and Outreach Enrollment, $12 million.
- BBA 2018, Section 50207, extended authority for these programs through September 30, 2019. For FY2018 and FY2019, BBA 2018 provides funding at the FY2017 funding level of $37.5 million annually in the following amounts: SHIPs, $13 million; AAAs, $7.5 million; ADRCs, $5 million; and the contract with the

National Center for Benefits and Outreach Enrollment, $12 million.

Current Status

Funding authorized under BBA 2018 for low-income outreach and assistance programs will expire after September 30, 2019. However, funds appropriated will be available for obligation until expended.

Patient-Centered Outcomes Research Trust Fund (IRC §9511 and §§4375-4377, SSA §1183); 26 U.S.C. §9511; 26 U.S.C. §§4375-4377; 42 U.S.C. §1320e-2

Background

SSA Section 1181 establishes the Patient-Centered Outcomes Research Institute (PCORI), which is responsible for coordinating and supporting comparative clinical effectiveness research. PCORI has entered into contracts with federal agencies, as well as with academic and private sector research entities for both the management of funding and conduct of research. PHSA Section 937 requires the Agency for Healthcare Research and Quality (AHRQ) to broadly disseminate research findings that are published by PCORI and other government-funded comparative effectiveness research entities.

IRC Section 9511 establishes the "Patient-Centered Outcomes Research Trust Fund" (PCORTF) to support the activities of PCORI and to fund activities under PHSA Section 937. It provides annual funding to the PCORTF over the period FY2010-FY2019 from the following three sources: (1) annual appropriations, (2) fees on health insurance and self-insured plans, and (3) transfers from the Medicare HI and SMI Trust Funds. SSA Section 1183 provides for the transfer of the required funds from the Medicare Trust Funds. Transfers to PCORTF from the Medicare HI and SMI Trust Funds are calculated based on the number of individuals entitled to benefits under Medicare Part A or enrolled in Medicare Part B. IRC Sections 4375-4377 impose the referenced fees on applicable health insurance policies and self-insured health plans and describe the method for their calculation.

For each of FY2011 through FY2019, IRC Section 9511 requires 80% of the PCORTF funds to be made available to PCORI, and the remaining 20% of funds to be transferred to the HHS Secretary for carrying out PHSA Section 937. Of the total amount transferred to HHS, 80% is to be distributed to AHRQ, with the remainder going to the Office of the Secretary (OS)/HHS.

Relevant Legislation

- ACA, Section 6301(e), provided the following amounts to the PCORTF: (1) $10 million for FY2010, (2) $50 million for FY2011, and (3) $150 million for each of FY2012 through FY2019. In addition, for each of FY2013 through FY2019, the section provided an amount equivalent to the net revenues from a new fee that the law imposed on health insurance policies and self-insured plans. For policy/plan years ending during FY2013, the fee equals $1 multiplied by the average number of covered lives. For policy/plan years ending during each subsequent fiscal year through FY2019, the fee equals $2 multiplied by the average number of covered lives. Finally, the section (in addition to ACA Section 6301(d)) provided for transfers to PCORTF from the Medicare Part A and Part B trust funds; these are generally calculated by multiplying the average number of individuals entitled to benefits under Medicare Part A, or enrolled in Medicare Part B, by $1 (for FY2013) or by $2 (for each of FY2014 through FY2019).

Current Status

Appropriated funds to PCORTF have not been enacted for FY2020 or subsequent fiscal years. Funds transferred to the HHS Secretary under IRC Section 9511 remain available until expended. No amounts shall be available for expenditure from the PCORTF after September 30, 2019, and any amounts in the Trust Fund after such date shall be transferred to the general fund of the Treasury.

SSA Title XIX: Medicaid

Protection for Recipients of Home and Community-Based Services against Spouse Impoverishment (SSA §1924; 42 U.S.C. 1296r-5)

Background

When determining financial eligibility for Medicaid-covered long-term services and supports (LTSS), there are specific rules under SSA Section 1924 for the treatment of a married couple's assets when one spouse needs long-term care provided in an institution, such as a nursing home. Commonly referred to as "spousal impoverishment rules," these rules attempt to equitably allocate income and assets to each spouse when determining Medicaid financial eligibility and are intended to prevent the impoverishment of the non-Medicaid spouse. For example, spousal impoverishment rules require state Medicaid programs to exempt all of a non-Medicaid spouse's income in his or her name from being considered available to the Medicaid spouse. Joint income of the couple is divided in half between the spouses, and the Medicaid spouse can transfer income to bring the non-Medicaid spouse up to certain income thresholds. Assets of the couple, regardless whose name they are in, are combined and then split in half. The non-Medicaid spouse can retain assets up to an asset threshold determined by the state within certain statutory parameters.[12] Prior to enactment of the ACA, spousal impoverishment rules applied only in situations where the Medicaid participant was receiving LTSS in an institution. States had the option to extend these protections to certain

[12] See Centers for Medicare & Medicaid Services (CMS), *2019 SSI and Spousal Impoverishment Standards,* at https://www.medicaid.gov/medicaid/eligibility/downloads/spousal-impoverishment/ssi-and-spousal-impoverishmentstandards.pdf.

home and community-based services (HCBS) participants under a Section 1915(c) waiver program.[13]

Beginning January 1, 2014, ACA Section 2404 temporarily substituted the definition of "institutionalized spouse" under SSA Section 1924(h)(1) to include application of these spousal impoverishment protections to all married individuals who are eligible for HCBS authorized under certain specified authorities. Thus, beginning January 1, 2014, for a five-year time period, the ACA required states to apply the spousal impoverishment rules to all married individuals who are eligible for HCBS under these specified authorities, not just those receiving institutional care.[14] This modified definition expired on December 31, 2018. The 116th Congress extended the authority for these protections and included a provision regarding state flexibility in the application of income or asset disregards for married individuals receiving certain HCBS.

Relevant Legislation

- ACA, Section 2404, required states to extend spousal impoverishment rules to certain beneficiaries receiving HCBS for a five-year period beginning on January 1, 2014.
- The Medicaid Extenders Act of 2019 (P.L. 116-3), Section 3, extended this provision through March 31, 2019.
- The Medicaid Services Investment and Accountability Act of 2019 (P.L. 116 16), Section 2, further extends this provision through September 30, 2019.

---

[13] These HCBS recipients are eligible under the "special home and community-based services waiver eligibility group" or "217 Group" in reference to the specific regulatory citation for this group at 42 CFR §435.217. Prior to Section 2404 of the ACA, states that chose to apply spousal impoverishment protections as an option for the 217 Group also had the option to treat married HCBS recipients in the 217 Group as institutionalized for the purposes of post-eligibility treatment of income (PETI) rules.

[14] States that cover the 217 Group must also apply the PETI rules.

Current Status

The authority for the extension of spousal impoverishment protections for certain Medicaid HCBS recipients will expire after September 30, 2019.

Additional Medicaid Funding for the Territories (SSA §1108; 42 U.S.C. §1308)

Background

Medicaid financing for the territories (i.e., America Samoa, Commonwealth of the Northern Mariana Islands, Guam, Puerto Rico, and the U.S. Virgin Islands) is different than the financing for the 50 states and the District of Columbia. Federal Medicaid funding to the states and the District of Columbia is open-ended, but the Medicaid programs in the territories are subject to annual federal capped funding.

The federal Medicaid funding for the territories comes from a few different sources. The permanent source of federal Medicaid funding for the territories is the annual capped funding. Since July 1, 2011, Medicaid funding for the territories has been supplemented by a few additional funding sources available for a limited time provided through the ACA; the Consolidated Appropriations Act, 2017 (P.L. 115-31); and BBA 2018. Prior to the availability of these additional Medicaid funding sources, all five territories typically exhausted their federal Medicaid funding prior to the end of the fiscal year.[15]

Relevant Legislation

- ACA, Section 2005, as modified by Section 10201, provided $6.3 billion in additional federal Medicaid funding to the territories available between July 1, 2011, and September 30, 2019.
- ACA, Section 1323, provided $1.0 billion in additional federal Medicaid funding to the territories that did not establish health

[15] For more information about Medicaid funding for the territories, see CRS In Focus IF11012, *Medicaid Funding for the Territories*.

insurance exchanges.[16] This funding is available January 1, 2014, through December 31, 2019.

- The Consolidated Appropriations Act, 2017 Division M, Title II, provided an additional $295.9 million in federal Medicaid funding to Puerto Rico available through September 30, 2019.
- BBA 2018, Division B, Subdivision 2, Title III, increased the federal Medicaid funding for Puerto Rico by $3.6 billion and the U.S. Virgin Islands by $106.9 million. This funding may be further increased by $1.2 billion for Puerto Rico and $35.6 million for U.S. Virgin Islands if certain conditions are met.[17] This funding is available January 1, 2018, through September 30, 2019.

Current Status

The $6.3 billion in additional Medicaid federal funding under ACA Section 2005 as modified and the additional funding provided to Puerto Rico and the U.S. Virgin Islands under the Consolidated Appropriations Act, 2017 and the BBA 2018 expire after September 30, 2019, and the $1.0 billion in ACA Section 1323 funding expires after December 31, 2019.

Public Health Service Act (PHSA) CY2019 Expiring Provisions

Community Health Center Fund (PHSA §330; 42 U.S.C. §254b-2(b)(1))

Background

The Community Health Center Fund (CHCF) provided mandatory funding for federal health centers authorized in PHSA Section 330. These

---

[16] Because none of the territories established exchanges, the territories all received additional federal Medicaid funds. Also, the provision specified that Puerto Rico receive $925 million, and the HHS Secretary distributed the remaining funding among the other four territories.

[17] The certain conditions are that the HHS Secretary needs to certify that each territory (i.e., Puerto Rico and U.S. Virgin Islands) has taken steps to (1) report reliable data to the Transformed-Medicaid Statistical Information System and (2) establish a Medicaid Fraud Control Unit.

centers are located in medically underserved areas and provide primary care, dental care, and other health and supportive services to individuals regardless of their ability to pay. The mandatory CHCF appropriations are provided in addition to discretionary funding for the program; however, the CHCF comprised more than 70% of health center programs' appropriations in FY2019.

Relevant Legislation

- ACA, Section 10503, established the CHCF and provided a total of $9.5 billion to the fund annually from FY2011 through FY2015, as follows: $1 billion for FY2011, $1.2 billion for FY2012, $1.5 billion for FY2013, $2.2 billion for FY2014, and $3.6 billion for FY2015. The ACA also provided $1.5 billion for health center construction and renovation for the period FY2011 through FY2015.
- MACRA, Section 221, provided $3.6 billion for each of FY2016 and FY2017 to the CHCF.
- An Act to amend the Homeland Security Act of 2002 to require the Secretary of Homeland Security to issue Department of Homeland Security-wide guidance and develop training programs as part of the Department of Homeland Security Blue Campaign, and for other purposes (P.L. 115-96), Section 3101(a), provided $550 million for the first and second quarters of FY2018 to the CHCF.
- BBA 2018, Section 50901, made a number of changes to the health center program replaced language that had provided two quarters of funding and provided $3.8 billion to the CHCF in FY2018 and $4.0 billion in FY2019.

Current Status

Appropriated funds for CHCF have been enacted for FY2019, but under current law no new funding is provided for FY2020 or subsequent fiscal years. Any unused portion of grants awarded for a given fiscal year prior to October 1, 2019, remains available until expended.

Special Diabetes Programs (PHSA §§330B and 330C; 42 U.S.C. §§254c-2(b) and 254c-3(b))

Background

The Special Diabetes Program for Type I Diabetes (PHSA Section 330B) provides funding for the National Institutes of Health to award grants for research into the prevention and cure of Type I diabetes. The Special Diabetes Program for Indians (PHSA Section 330C) provides funding for the Indian Health Service (IHS) to award grants for services related to the prevention and treatment of diabetes for American Indians and Alaska Natives who receive services at IHSfunded facilities.

Relevant Legislation

- The Balanced Budget Act of 1997 (BBA 97; P.L. 105-33), Sections 4921 and 4922, established the two special diabetes programs and transferred $30 million annually from CHIP funds to each program from FY1998 through FY2002.
- The Medicare, Medicaid, and SCHIP Benefits Improvement and Protection Act of 2000 (BIPA 2000; P.L. 106-554), Section 931, increased each program's annual appropriations to $70 million for FY2001 through FY2002 and provided $100 million for FY2003.
- P.L. 107-360, Section 1, increased each program's annual appropriations to $150 million and provided funds from FY2004 through FY2008.
- MMSEA, Section 302, provided $150 million through FY2009.
- MIPPA, Section 303, provided $150 million through FY2011.
- MMEA, Section 112, provided $150 million through FY2013.
- ATRA, Section 625, provided $150 million through FY2014.
- PAMA, Section 204, provided of $150 million through FY2015.
- MACRA, Section 213, provided $150 million through FY2017.

- Disaster Tax Relief and Airport and Airway Extension Act of 2017 (P.L. 115- 63), Section 301(b), provided $37.5 million for first quarter of FY2018 for the Special Diabetes Program for Indians (Note: it did not provide funding for the Special Diabetes Program for Type I Diabetes.)
- P.L. 115-96, Section 3102, provided $37.5 million for the second quarter for the Special Diabetes Program for Indians and provided $37.5 million for the first and second quarters of FY2018 for the Special Diabetes Program for Type I Diabetes.
- BBA 2018, Section 50902, replaced language that had provided funding for the first and second quarters of FY2018 to provide $150 million for each program in FY2018 and FY2019.

Current Status

Appropriated funds for the two special diabetes programs have been enacted for FY2019, but under current law no new funding is provided for FY2020 or subsequent fiscal years. Any unused portion of grants awarded for a given fiscal year prior to October 1, 2019, remains available until expended.

National Health Service Corps Appropriations (PHSA §338H; 42 U.S.C. §254b-2(b)(2))

Background

The National Health Service Corps (NHSC) provides scholarships and loan repayments to certain health professionals in exchange for providing care in a health professional shortage area for a period of time that varies based on the length of the scholarship or the number of years of loan repayment received. The NHSC receives mandatory funding from the CHCF through PHSA Title III. The NHSC also received discretionary appropriations in FY2011. Between FY2012 and FY2017, the program did not receive discretionary appropriations.

Beginning in FY2018 and continuing in FY2019, the program received discretionary appropriations, primarily to expand the number and type of substance abuse providers participating in the NHSC. The mandatory funding from the CHCF represents more nearly three-quarters of the program's funding in both FY2018 and FY2019.

Relevant Legislation

- ACA, Section 10503, funded $1.5 billion to support the NHSC annually from FY2011 through FY2015, as follows: $290 million for FY2011, $295 million for FY2012, $300 million for FY2013, $305 million for FY2014, and $310 million for FY2015. Funds are to remain available until expended.
- MACRA, Section 221, funded $310 million for each of FY2016 and FY2017 for the NHSC.
- P.L. 115-96, Section 3101(b), funded $65 million for the first and second quarters of FY2018 for the NHSC.
- BBA 2018, Section 50901(c), replaced language that had provided two-quarters of funding and funded $310 million for each of FY2018 and FY2019 for the NHSC.

Current Status

Appropriated funds for CHCF funds have been enacted for FY2019, but under current law no new funding is provided for FY2020 or subsequent fiscal years. Any unused portion of grants awarded for a given fiscal year prior to October 1, 2019, remains available until expended.

Teaching Health Centers (PHSA §340H; 42 U.S.C. §256h)

Background

The Teaching Health Center program provides direct and indirect graduate medical education (GME) payments to support medical and dental residents training at qualified teaching health centers (i.e., outpatient health care facilities that provide care to underserved patients).

Relevant Legislation

- ACA, Section 5508(a), established the Teaching Health Center program and provided $230 million for direct and indirect GME payments for the period of FY2011 through FY2015.
- MACRA, Section 221, provided $60 million for each of FY2016 and FY2017 for direct and indirect GME payments for teaching health centers.
- Disaster Tax Relief and Airport and Airway Extension Act of 2017, Section 301(a), provided $15 million for the first quarter of FY2018 for direct and indirect GME payments for teaching health centers.
- P.L. 115-96, Section 3101(c), struck the first quarter of funding and provided $30 million for the first and second quarters of FY2018 for direct and indirect GME payments for teaching health centers. It also limited the amount of funding that could be used for administrative purposes.
- BBA 2018, Section 50901(d), made a number of changes to the Teaching Health Center program and replaced language that had provided two-quarters of funding and provided $126.5 million for each of FY2018 and FY2019 for direct and indirect GME payments for teaching health centers.

Current Status

Appropriated funds for Teaching Health Center GME payments have been enacted for FY2019. Under current law no new funding is provided for FY2020 or subsequent fiscal years.

OTHER CY2019 EXPIRING PROVISIONS

Health Coverage Tax Credit (IRC §35; 26 U.S.C. §35)

Background

The Health Coverage Tax Credit (HCTC) subsidizes 72.5% of the cost of *qualified health insurance* for eligible taxpayers and their family members. Potential eligibility for the HCTC is limited to two groups of taxpayers. One group is composed of individuals eligible for Trade Adjustment Assistance (TAA) allowances because they experienced qualifying job losses. The other group consists of individuals whose defined-benefit pension plans were taken over by the Pension Benefit Guaranty Corporation because of financial difficulties. HCTC-eligible individuals are allowed to receive the tax credit only if they either cannot enroll in certain other health coverage (e.g., Medicaid) or are not eligible for other specified coverage (e.g., Medicare Part A). To claim the HCTC, eligible taxpayers must have qualified health insurance (specific categories of coverage, as specified in statute). The credit is financed through a permanent appropriation under 31 U.S.C. §1324(b)(2); therefore, the financing of the HCTC is not subject to the annual appropriations process.

Relevant Legislation

- The Trade Act of 2002 (P.L. 107-210), Sections 201-203, authorized the Health Coverage Tax Credit, specified the eligibility criteria for claiming the credit, and made conforming amendment to the *U.S. Code* for purposes of financing the credit.
- The American Recovery and Reinvestment Act of 2009 (ARRA, P.L. 111-5), Part VI: TAA Health Coverage Improvement Act of 2009 expanded eligibility for and subsidy of the HCTC including retroactive amendments, and provided $80 million for FY2009 and FY2010 to implement the enacted changes to the HCTC.

- The Trade Adjustment Assistance Extension Act of 2011 (P.L. 112-40), Section 241, established a sunset date of before January 1, 2014.
- The Trade Preferences Extension Act of 2015 (P.L. 114-27), Section 407, retroactively reauthorized the HCTC and established a new sunset date of before January 1, 2020.

Current Status

Authorization for the HCTC is scheduled to expire after December 31, 2019.

Annual Fee on Health Insurance Providers (ACA §9010)

Background

An annual fee is imposed on certain health insurance issuers. The aggregate fee is set at $8.0 billion in CY2014, $11.3 billion in CY2015 and CY2016, $13.9 billion in CY2017, and $14.3 billion in CY2018. After CY2018, the fee is indexed to the annual rate of U.S. premium growth. The fee is based on net health care premiums written by covered issuers during the year prior to the year in which payment is due. Each year, the Internal Revenue Service calculates the fee on covered issuers based on (1) their net premiums written in the previous calendar year as a share of total net premiums written by all covered issuers and (2) their dollar value of business. Covered issuers are not subject to the fee on their first $25 million of net premiums written. The fee is imposed on 50% of net premiums above $25 million and up to $50 million and on 100% of net premiums in excess of $50 million.

Relevant Legislation

- ACA, Section 9010, established the annual fee on certain health insurance issuers. The fee became effective for CY2014.

- The Consolidated Appropriations Act, 2016 (P.L. 114-113), Division P, Title II, Section 201, suspended collection of the fee for CY2017.
- Making further continuing appropriations for the fiscal year ending September 30, 2018, and for other purposes (P.L. 115-120), Section 4003, suspended collection of the fee for CY2019.

Current Status

The moratorium on the collection of the fee is to end after CY2019, meaning covered entities are scheduled to be subject to the fee again beginning in CY2020.

Excise Tax on Medical Device Manufacturers (26 U.S.C. §4191)

Background

An excise tax is imposed on the sale of certain medical devices. For the purposes of the tax, a "medical device" is defined by the Federal Food, Drug, and Cosmetic Act (21 U.S.C. §321(h)) and pertains to devices "intended for humans." Congress exempted eyeglasses, contact lenses, and hearing aids from the tax and any other medical device determined by the Secretary of the Treasury to be of the type that is "generally purchased by the general public at retail for individual use." The tax is equal to 2.3% of the device's sales price and generally is imposed on the manufacturer or importer of the device.

Relevant Legislation

- The Health Care and Education Reconciliation Act of 2010 (HCERA; P.L. 111-152), Section 1405, created the excise tax on medical device manufacturers starting in CY2013.
- The Consolidated Appropriations Act, 2016, Division Q, Title I, Subtitle C, Part 2, Section 174, suspended imposition of the tax for CY2016 and CY2017.

- Making further continuing appropriations for the fiscal year ending September 30, 2018, and for other purposes (P.L. 115-120), Section 4001, extended the suspension of the imposition of the tax for CY2018 and CY2019.

Current Status

The suspension of the tax is to end after CY2019, meaning the tax is to apply to sales of medical devices again beginning in CY2020.

CY2017 AND CY2018 EXPIRED PROVISIONS

SSA Title XVIII: Medicare

Temporary Exception for Certain Severe Wound Discharges from Application of the Medicare Site Neutral Payment for Certain Long Term Care Hospitals (SSA §1886(m)(6)(E) and (G); 42 U.S.C. §1395ww(m)(6)(E) and (G))

Background

Medicare pays LTCHs for inpatient hospital care under the LTCH PPS, which is typically higher than payments for inpatient hospital care under the IPPS. Effective for cost-reporting periods beginning in FY2016, LTCHS are paid the LTCH PPS rate for patients that meet one of the following two criteria: (1) had a prior three-day intensive-care-unit stay at a hospital paid under the IPPS immediately preceding the LTCH stay or (2) is assigned to an LTCH PPS case-mix group that is based on the receipt of ventilator services for at least 96 hours and had a prior hospital stay at a hospital paid under the IPPS immediately preceding the LTCH stay. Discharges involving patients who have a principal diagnosis relating to a psychiatric diagnosis or rehabilitation do not qualify for the LTCH PPS rate. For LTCH discharges that did not qualify for the LTCH PPS based on these criteria, a site neutral payment rate is being phased-in for cost-reporting periods beginning FY2016 through FY2019. Subsequent legislation provided for other criteria to temporarily receive payment under the LTCH PPS. See section "Temporary Extension of Long-Term Care Hospital (LTCH) Site Neutral Payment Policy Transition Period (SSA §1886(m)(6)(B)(i); 42 U.S.C. §1395ww(m)(6)(B)(i))" for details related to site neutral payment.

Relevant Legislation

- The Consolidated Appropriations Act, 2016, Division H, Title II, Section 231, provided an additional temporary criterion for payment under the LTCH PPS for discharges before January 1, 2017. Specifically, the LTCH PPS rate would apply to an LTCH discharge if all three of the following are satisfied: (1) the LTCH is a grandfathered hospital-within-hospital; (2) the LTCH is located in a rural area; and (3) the patient discharged has a severe wound—defined as a stage 3 or 4 wound, unstageable wound, nonhealing surgical wound, infected wound, fistula, osteomyelitis, or wound with morbid obesity.
- Cures Act, Division C, Section 15010, reinstated, after a lapse period and with some modifications, the temporary criterion for payment under the LTCH PPS related to certain spinal cord conditions for discharges occurring in cost-reporting period beginning during FY2018. The reinstated temporary criterion, similar to the Consolidated Appropriations Act of 2016 criterion, applies only to a grandfathered hospital-within-hospital. It eliminates the requirement from Consolidated Appropriations Act of 2016 that an LTCH be located in a rural area and narrows the definition of a severe wound that was used in Consolidated Appropriations Act of 2016. In addition, unlike the Consolidated Appropriations Act of 2016 criterion, only discharges associated with diagnosis-related groups relating to cellulitis or osteomyelitis are eligible for the reinstated temporary criterion.

Current Status

The temporary criterion for certain severe wound discharges for payment under the LTCH PPS expired for discharges in cost-reporting periods beginning during FY2019 and subsequent years.

Exclusion of ASC Physicians from the Medicare Meaningful Use Payment Adjustment (SSA §1848(a)(7)(D); 42 U.S.C. §1395w–4(a)(7)(D))

Background

Congress has passed several bills to promote the widespread adoption of health information technology (HIT) and to support the electronic sharing of clinical data among hospitals, physicians, and other health care stakeholders. HIT encompasses interoperable electronic health records (EHRs)—including computerized systems to order tests and medications, and support systems to aid clinical decision making—and the development of a national health information network to permit the secure exchange of electronic health information among providers.

Relevant Legislation

- ARRA, Section 4101, which incorporated the Health Information Technology for Economic and Clinical Health Act (HITECH), authorized Medicare and Medicaid incentive payments to acute-care hospitals and physicians who attest to being meaningful users of certified EHR technology. The law instructed the HHS Secretary to make the measures of "meaningful use" more stringent over time, which CMS has done in stages. Beginning in CY2015, hospitals and physicians that were or are not meaningful EHR users are subject to a Medicare payment adjustment (i.e., penalty) unless they qualify for a hardship exception.
- Cures Act, Section 16003, exempted physicians who furnish "substantially all" of their services to patients in ambulatory surgery centers from a meaningful use payment penalty in CY2017

and CY2018 because physicians who provide services to beneficiaries in ASCs faced additional difficulties in meeting some of the meaningful use criteria.

Current Status

The exemption as specified in the Cures Act expired December 31, 2018. Current law states that this exemption is to sunset "as of the first year that begins more than 3 years after the date on which the Secretary determines, through notice and comment rulemaking, that certified EHR technology applicable to the ambulatory surgical center setting is available." This has yet to occur.

Delay in Authority to Terminate Contracts for Medicare Advantage (MA) Plans Failing to Achieve Minimum Quality Ratings (SSA §1857; 42 U.S.C. §1395w-27)

Background

Under Medicare Advantage (Medicare Part C, or MA) CMS pays private health plans a per-enrollee amount to provide all Medicare-covered benefits (except hospice) to beneficiaries who enroll in their plan. SSA Section 1853(o)(4) requires the HHS Secretary to use a five-star quality rating system to adjust maximum possible payments to high-performing MA plans. High star quality also results in an increase in an MA organization's rebate if its contract bid is less than the maximum amount that Medicare will pay. In addition, the five-star quality ratings are publicly reported and can be used by beneficiaries when considering which MA, Part D, or Medicare Advantage-Prescription Drug (MA-PD) plan to enroll in.

The Social Security Act authorizes the HHS Secretary to terminate a contract with an MA organization or a Perscription Drug Plan (PDP) if the HHS Secretary determines that the MA organization or PDP has failed substantially to carry out the contract, is carrying out the contract in a manner inconsistent with the efficient and effective administration of the Medicare program, or no longer meets the applicable Medicare program conditions.[18] CMS amended its regulations in 2012 to include a ground for contract termination relating to an MA organization's or a PDP's rating under the five-star system. Specifically, under the regulation, CMS may terminate a contract with an MA organization or a PDP if the plan receives a "summary plan rating of less than 3 stars for 3 consecutive contract years."[19] The regulation applies to plan ratings issued by CMS after September 1, 2012. CMS has terminated some MA organizations' contracts on this basis.

Relevant Legislation

- Cures Act, Division C, Section 17001: through the end of plan year 2018, the HHS Secretary is prohibited from terminating an MA organization's contract (or Part D contract) solely because the contract failed to achieve a minimum quality rating under the five-star rating system.

Current Status

The HHS Secretary has the authority to terminate an organization's MA or Part D contract based solely on the organization's receipt of a Part C or Part D summary rating of less than three stars for three consecutive contract years. The Secretary issued a memorandum to MA plans indicating that the first star rating released after December 2018 is the first that could count toward termination. Star ratings are released in the fall of one year, displayed for beneficiary use the next year, and then used for payment purposes the following year. As such, the CY2020 rates (released fall CY2019 and used for payment purposes in CY2021) are the first that could apply toward potential termination. The soonest possible effective date for a CMS termination of an MA contract under this policy would be December 31, 2022.

---

[18] SSA §1857(c)(2) (contract termination authority under Medicare Advantage) and §1860D-12(b)(3)(B) (contract termination authority under Medicare Part D).

[19] 42 C.F. R. §§422.510(a)(4)(xi), 423.509(a)(4)(x) CMS, "Medicare Program; Changes to the Medicare Advantage and the Medicare Prescription Drug Benefit Programs for Contract Year 2013 and Other Changes" *77 Federal Register* 22072-22175, April 12, 2012.

Other Medicare Provisions

Delay in Applying the 25% Patient Threshold Payment Adjustment for Long-Term Care Hospitals (MMSEA §114(c); 42 U.S.C. §1395ww note)

Background

LTCHs generally treat patients who have been discharged from acute-care hospitals but require prolonged inpatient hospital care due to their medical conditions. LTCH patients have an average length of inpatient stay longer than 25 days. LTCHs can be (1) freestanding—a hospital generally not integrated with any other hospital; (2) co-located with another hospital, either located in the same building as another hospital or in a separate building on the hospital's campus; or (3) a satellite facility of an LTCH—a separately located facility (which may be co-located with another hospital) that operates as part of the LTCH.

Beginning in FY2005, CMS implemented a new Medicare payment regulation for LTCHs that are co-located with other hospitals and LTCH satellite facilities to limit inappropriate patient shifting driven by financial rather than clinical considerations. Under the new policy, if such an LTCH received more than 25% of its Medicare patients from any single referring hospital, the LTCH is paid the lower of the LTCH PPS or the IPPS payment for discharges that exceeded the threshold.

Beginning in FY2008, CMS expanded the 25% patient threshold adjustment policy to include all LTCHs.

Relevant Legislation

- MMSEA, Section 114(c)(1), delayed the application of CMS's 25% patient threshold adjustment for freestanding LTCHs and "grandfathered hospitalswithin-hospitals" LTCHs for three years from the enactment of MMSEA (December 29, 2007). MMSEA Section 114(c)(2) delayed the application of CMS's 25% patient threshold adjustment for LTCHs or satellite facilities co-located with another hospital if (1) LTCHs or satellite facilities located in a rural area or co-located with an urban single or Metropolitan Statistical Area (MSA) dominant hospital receive no more than 75% of their Medicare inpatients from such co-located hospitals or (2) other LTCHs or satellite facilities co-located with another hospital receive no more than 50% of their Medicare inpatients from such co-located hospitals.

- ARRA, Section 4302(a), modified the beginning of the delays in MMSEA Sections 114(c)(1) and 114(c)(2) from the date of enactment of MMSEA (December 29, 2007) to July 1, 2007. This section also modified the end date for the delay under MMSEA Section 114(c)(2) (LTCHs co-located with another hospital) from three years from the date of enactment to three years from October 1, 2007 (or July 1, 2007, in the case of a satellite facility described in 42 C.F.R. §412.22(h)(3)(i)). In addition, ARRA Section 4302(a) modified the delay under MMSEA Section 114(c)(1) to include LTCHs or satellite facilities that, as of the date of enactment under MMSEA, were co-located with a provider-based off-campus location of an IPPS hospital that did not provide services payable under the IPPS at the off-campus location.
- ACA, Section 3106, extended the delay of the 25% patient threshold adjustment two additional years.
- PSRA, Section 1206(b)(1), extended the delay of the 25% patient threshold adjustment four additional years to expire after June 30, 2016 (or after September 30, 2016, for certain LTCHs co-located with another hospital).
- Cures Act, Division C, Section 15006, delayed the 25% patient threshold adjustment for discharges occurring October 1, 2016, through September 30, 2017. This provision reinstated the PSRA delay that expired after June 30, 2016 (and extended the PSRA delay that expired after September 30, 2016, for certain LTCHs co-located with another hospital).

Current Status

The statutory delay in CMS applying the 25% patient threshold adjustment to LTCHs expired after September 30, 2017. However, the HHS Secretary extended the delay through FY2018 and eliminated it beginning FY2019 through rulemaking.[20]

Long-Term Care Hospital Moratoria (MMSEA §114(d); 42 U.S.C. §1395ww note)

Background

Under Medicare, LTCHs were exempt from the IPPS when it was established in 1983. Instead, LTCHs were paid on a reasonable-cost basis subject to certain limits established by the Tax Equity and Fiscal Responsibility Act of 1982 (TEFRA; P.L. 97-248). Under the Balanced Budget Refinement Act of 1999 (BBRA 99; P.L. 106-113), the LTCH PPS was established, which provides a per-discharge payment based on the average costs and patient mix of LTCHs. The LTCH PPS typically provides higher Medicare payment rates for inpatient hospital care than the IPPS.

The rapid increase in both the number of LTCHs and LTCH payments led to enactment of a temporary moratorium on the development of new LTCHs and a moratorium on new LTCH beds, with certain exceptions.

Relevant Legislation

- MMSEA, Section 114(d), established a three-year moratorium from the date of enactment (December 29, 2007) on the development of new LTCHs, with exceptions for (1) LTCHs that

[20] CMS, "Medicare Program; Hospital Inpatient Prospective Payment Systems for Acute Care Hospitals and the Long-Term Care Hospital Prospective Payment System and Policy Changes and Fiscal Year 2019 Rates; Quality Reporting Requirements for Specific Providers; Medicare and Medicaid Electronic Health Record (EHR) Incentive Programs (Promoting Interoperability Programs) Requirements for Eligible Hospitals, Critical Access Hospitals, and Eligible Professionals; Medicare Cost Reporting Requirements; and Physician Certification and Recertification of Claims", 83 *Federal Register* 41144, August 17, 2018, see pages 41532-41533.

began their qualifying period for Medicare reimbursement before the enactment of MMSEA; (2) LTCHs that had a binding written agreement before the enactment of MMSEA for the actual construction, renovation, lease, or demolition of an LTCH, and had expended at least 10% of the estimated cost of the project (or $2.5 million, if less); and (3) LTCHs that had obtained an approved certificate of need in a state where one is required on or before the date of enactment of MMSEA. MMSEA Section 114(d) also established a three-year moratorium from the date of enactment (December 29, 2007) on the increase in beds in existing LTCHs, with exceptions for (1) LTCHs located in a state where there is only one other LTCH and (2) LTCHs that request an increase in beds following the closure or decrease in the number of beds of another LTCH in the state.

- ARRA, Section 4302, amended the three-year moratorium on the increase in beds in existing LTCHs by providing an exception to LTCHs that had obtained a certificate of need for such an increase in LTCH beds on or after April 1, 2005, and before the enactment of MMSEA.
- ACA, Section 3106(b), extended the moratoria established under MMSEA an additional two years (expiring after December 29, 2012).
- PSRA, Section 1206(b)(2), reinstated the moratoria under MMSEA beginning January 1, 2015, and expiring after September 30, 2017; however, PSRA did not allow any exceptions to the reinstated moratoria.
- PAMA, Section 112(b), amended the moratoria reinstated by PSRA to begin with enactment of PSRA (December 26, 2013) rather than January 1, 2015. Further, this section provided the same exceptions on the development of new LTCHs that had been provided under MMSEA but did not provide exceptions for the increase in LTCH beds.

- Cures Act, Division C, Section 15004, reinstated the exception to the moratorium on the increase in LTCH beds effective as if it had been enacted by PAMA, April 1, 2014, to coincide with the previously reinstated exception for new LTCHs.

Current Status

The moratorium on the development of new LTCHs and on the increase of beds in existing LTCHs expired as of September 30, 2017.

Extension of Enforcement Instruction on Supervision Requirements for Outpatient Therapeutic Services in Critical Access and Small Rural Hospitals

Background

The 2009 Outpatient Prospective Payment System (OPPS) final rule required that therapeutic hospital outpatient services be furnished under the direct supervision of a physician.[21] However, beginning in CY2010, CMS instructed its contractors not to evaluate or enforce the supervision requirements for therapeutic services provided to outpatients in critical access hospitals (CAHs). CMS extended this non-enforcement instruction for CY2011 and expanded it to include small rural hospitals with 100 or fewer beds. Subsequently, CMS extended the instruction for CY2012 and CY2013, The non-enforcement instruction has been extended several more times through legislation and rules.

Relevant Legislation

- An Act to Provide for the Extension of the Enforcement Instruction on Supervision Requirements for Outpatient Therapeutic Services in Critical Access and Small Rural Hospitals

[21] CMS, "Medicare Program: Changes to the Hospital Outpatient Prospective Payment System and CY 2010 Payment Rates; Changes to the Ambulatory Surgical Center Payment System and CY 2010 Payment Rates," 74 *Federal Register* 60315-60983, November 20, 2009.

Through 2014 (P.L. 113-198), required the HHS Secretary to extend the non-enforcement instruction through CY2014.

- An Act to Provide for the Extension of the Enforcement Instruction on Supervision Requirements for Outpatient Therapeutic Services in Critical Access and Small Rural Hospitals Through 2015 (P.L. 114-112), required the HHS Secretary to extend the non-enforcement instruction through CY2015.
- Cures Act, Section 16004, extended the non-enforcement instruction through CY2016.
- BBA 2018, Section 51007, extended the non-enforcement instruction through CY2017 retroactively.

Current Status

Although the non-enforcement instruction has statutorily expired, the CY2018 OPPS/ Ambulatory Surgery Center (ASC) final rule with comment period re-established the nonenforcement policy beginning on January 1, 2018, and extended the instruction through December 31, 2019.[22]

APPENDIX A. DEMONSTRATION PROJECTS AND PILOT PROGRAMS

This appendix lists selected health care-related demonstration projects and pilot programs that are scheduled to expire during the first session of the 116th Congress (i.e., during calendar year [CY] 2019).

The expiring demonstration projects and pilot programs listed below have portions of law that are time-limited and will lapse once a statutory deadline is reached, absent further legislative action.

---

[22] CMS, "Medicare Program: Hospital Outpatient Prospective Payment and Ambulatory Surgical Center Payment Systems and Quality Reporting Programs," 82 *Federal Register* 52356, November 11, 2017.

Table A-1. Demonstration projects and pilot programs expiring in the 116th Congress, First Session (CY2019)

Expires After	Health Care Related Program	Provision		Contact
6/30/2019[a]	Medicaid/ Other	Demonstration to Improve Community Behavioral Health Clinics	PAMA §223(f) 42 U.S.C. §1396a	Alison Mitchell
9/30/2019	Medicaid	Money Follows the Person Rebalancing Demonstration[b]	DRA §6071 42 U.S.C. §1396a note	Kirsten Colello
9/30/2019	Other	Demonstration Projects to Address Health Professions Workforce Needs[c]	SSA §2008(c) 42 U.S.C. §1397g[d]	Elayne Heisler

Source: Congressional Research Service.

Notes: CY = Calendar Year, DRA = Deficit Reduction Act of 2005, PAMA = Protecting Access to Medicare Act of 2014, SSA = Social Security Act, U.S.C. = *U.S. Code*.

[a]The expiration date of Demonstration to Improve Community Behavioral Health Clinics was amended in the Medicaid Services Investment and Accountability Act of 2019 (P.L. 116-16), and the expiration date is effectively June 30, 2019. For more information, see https://www.samhsa.gov/section-223.

[b]Extended most recently in Section 2 of the Medicaid Extenders Act of 2019 (P.L. 116-3; additional funding provided under Section 5 of the Medicaid Services Investment and Accountability Act of 2019 (P.L. 116-16). For more information, see https://www.medicaid.gov/medicaid/ltss/money-follows-the-person/index.html.

[c]For more information, see https://www.acf.hhs.gov/ofa/ programs/hpog.

[d]Authorization for this program is included in SSA §2008(a), and mandatory appropriations for the program are included in SSA §2008(c).

The expiring demonstration projects and pilot programs included here are those related to Medicare, Medicaid, the State Children's Health Insurance Program (CHIP), and private health insurance programs and activities.[23]

---

[23] Section 3021 of the Patient Protection and Affordable Care Act (ACA; P.L. 111-148, as amended) amended Title XI of the Social Security Act (SSA) to establish the Center for Medicare and Medicaid Innovation (CMMI). CMMI is authorized to test payment and service delivery models to improve the quality of care and/or reduce spending. For more information on the Center for Medicare and Medicaid Innovation (CMMI), see

This appendix also includes other health care-related demonstration projects and pilot programs that were enacted in the Patient Protection and Affordable Care Act (ACA; P.L. 111-148) or last extended under the Bipartisan Budget Act of 2018 (BBA 2018; P.L. 115-123). In addition, this appendix lists health care-related demonstration projects and pilot programs within the same scope that expired during the 115th Congress (i.e., during CY2017 or CY2018).

Although every attempt to be comprehensive has been made, we cannot guarantee that every relevant demonstration project and pilot program is included here.

Table A-1, lists the relevant demonstration projects and pilot programs that are scheduled to expire in 2019. Table A-2 lists the relevant provisions that expired during 2018 or 2017

Table A-2. Demonstration projects and pilot programs that expired in the 115th Congress

Expired After	Health Care Related Program	Provision		Contact
3/23/2017	Other	Demonstration Program to Increase Access to Dental Health Care Services[a]	PHSA §340G-1 42 U.S.C. §256g-1	Elayne Heisler

Source: Congressional Research Service.

Notes: CY = Calendar Year, PHSA = Public Health Service Act, U.S.C. = *U.S. Code*.

[a]A provision prohibiting the Health Resources and Services Administration from funding this demonstration program has been included in the Departments of Labor, Health and Human Services, Education, and Related Agencies appropriations act for each of FY2011-FY2016 and for FY2017 appropriations under continuing resolutions (P.L. 114-223 and P.L. 114-254).

https://innovation.cms.gov/, and CMS, CMMI, *Report to Congress: December 2016,* at https://innovation.cms.gov/Files/reports/rtc-2016.pdf.

Appendix B. Laws That Created, Modified, or Extended Current Health Care-Related Expiring Provisions

Table B-1. Laws That Created, Modified, or Extended Current Health Care-Related Expiring Provisions

P.L. Number	Acronym	Act Title
P.L. 97-248	TEFRA	Tax Equity and Fiscal Responsibility Act of 1982
P.L. 101-239	—	Omnibus Budget Reconciliation Act of 1989
P.L. 101-508	OBRA 90	Omnibus Budget Reconciliation Act of 1990
P.L. 104-191	HIPPA	Health Insurance Portability and Protection Act of 1996
P.L. 104-193	PRWORA	Personal Responsibility and Work Opportunity Reconciliation Act of 1996
P.L. 105-33	BBA 97	Balanced Budget Act of 1997
P.L. 106-113	BBRA 99	Balanced Budget Refinement Act of 1999
P.L. 106-554	BIPA 2000	Medicare, Medicaid, and SCHIP Benefits Improvement and Protection Act of 2000
P.L. 107-360	—	An Act to Amend the Public Health Service Act with Respect to Special Diabetes Programs for Type 1 Diabetes and Indians
P.L. 108-40	WREA 2003	Welfare Reform Extension Act of 2003
P.L. 108-74	—	State Children's Health Insurance Program Allotments Extension Act
P.L. 108-89	—	An Act to Extend the Temporary Assistance for Needy Families Block Grant Program, and Certain Tax and Trade Programs, and For Other Purposes
P.L. 108-173	MMA	Medicare Prescription Drug, Improvement, and Modernization Act of 2003a
P.L. 108-210	WREA 2004	Welfare Reform Extension Act of 2004
P.L. 108-262	—	TANF and Related Programs Continuation Act of 2004
P.L. 108-308	—	Welfare Reform Extension Act, Part VIII
P.L. 109-4	WREA 2005	Welfare Reform Extension Act of 2005
P.L. 109-19	—	TANF Extension Act of 2005
P.L. 109-91	—	QI, TMA, and Abstinence Programs Extension and Hurricane Katrina Unemployment Relief Act of 2005
P.L. 109-171	DRA	Deficit Reduction Act of 2005
P.L. 109-432	TRHCA	Tax Relief and Health Care Act of 2006
P.L. 109-482	—	National Institutes of Health Reform Act of 2006
P.L. 110-48	—	An Act to Provide for the Extension of Transitional Medical Assistance, and Other Provisions
P.L. 110-90	—	TMA, Abstinence Education, and QI Programs Extension Act of 2007

P.L. Number	Acronym	Act Title
P.L. 110-92	—	Making Continuing Appropriations for the Fiscal Year 2008, and for Other Purposes
P.L. 110-116	—	Department of Defense Appropriations Act of 2008
P.L. 110-137	—	Making Further Continuing Appropriations for the Fiscal Year 2008, and for Other Purposes.
P.L. 110-149	—	Making Further Continuing Appropriations for the Fiscal Year 2008, and for Other Purposes.
P.L. 110-173	MMSEA	Medicare, Medicaid, and SCHIP Extension Act of 2007b
P.L. 110-275	MIPPA	Medicare Improvements for Patients and Providers Act of 2008c
P.L. 111-3	CHIPRA	Children's Health Insurance Program Reauthorization Act of 2009d
P.L. 111-5	ARRA	American Recovery and Reinvestment Act of 2009e
P.L. 111-148	ACA	Patient Protection and Affordable Care Act of 2010f
P.L. 111-152	HCERA	Health Care and Education Reconciliation Act of 2010g
P.L. 111-309	MMEA	Medicare and Medicaid Extenders Act of 2010
P.L. 112-78	TPTCCA	Temporary Payroll Tax Cut Continuation Act of 2011
P.L. 112-96	MCTRJCA	Middle Class Tax Relief and Job Creation Act of 2012
P.L. 112-240	ATRA	American Taxpayer Relief Act of 2012h
P.L. 113-67	BBA 13/PSRA	Continuing Appropriations Resolution of 2014, which includes Division A, the Bipartisan Budget Act of 2013, and Division B, the Pathway for SGR Reform Act of 2013
P.L. 113-93	PAMA	Protecting Access to Medicare Act of 2014
P.L. 113-198	—	An Act to Provide for the Extension of the Enforcement Instruction on Supervision Requirements for Outpatient Therapeutic Services in Critical Access and Small Rural Hospitals Through 2014
P.L. 114-10	MACRA	Medicare Access and CHIP Reauthorization Act of 2015i
P.L. 114-112	—	An Act to Provide for the Extension of the Enforcement Instruction on Supervision Requirements for Outpatient Therapeutic Services in Critical Access and Small Rural Hospitals Through 2015
P.L. 114-113	—	Consolidated Appropriations Act of 2016
P.L. 114-115	PAMPA	Patient Access and Medicare Protection Act
P.L. 114-255	Cures Act	The 21st Century Cures Act
P.L. 115-31	—	Consolidated Appropriations Act, 2017
P.L. 115-63	—	Disaster Tax Relief and Airport and Airway Extension Act of 2017
P.L. 115-96	—	An Act to amend the Homeland Security Act of 2002 to require the Secretary of Homeland Security to issue Department of Homeland Security-wide guidance and develop training programs as part of the Department of Homeland Security Blue Campaign, and for other purposes

Table B-1. (Continued)

P.L. Number	Acronym	Act Title
P.L. 115-120	—	Making Further Continuing Appropriations for the Fiscal Year Ending September 30, 2018, and for Other Purposes.
P.L. 115-123	BBA 2018	Bipartisan Budget Act of 2018
P.L. 116-3	—	Medicaid Extenders Act of 2019
P.L. 116-16	—	Medicaid Services Investment and Accountability Act of 2019

Source: Congressional Research Service (CRS).

Notes:

a. See CRS Report RL31966, Overview of the Medicare Prescription Drug, Improvement, and Modernization Act of 2003, and CRS Report RL32005, Medicare Fee-for-Service Modifications and Medicaid Provisions of H.R. 1 as Enacted.

b. See CRS Report RL34360, P.L. 110-173: Provisions in the Medicare, Medicaid, and SCHIP Extension Act of 2007.

c. See CRS Report RL34592, P.L. 110-275: The Medicare Improvements for Patients and Providers Act of 2008.

d. See CRS Report R40226, P.L. 111-3: The Children's Health Insurance Program Reauthorization Act of 2009.

e. The Health Information Technology for Economic and Clinical Health Act was incorporated into ARRA. A description of the Medicare provisions in that bill can be found in CRS Report R40161, The Health Information Technology for Economic and Clinical Health (HITECH) Act.

f. See CRS Report R41196, Medicare Provisions in the Patient Protection and Affordable Care Act (PPACA): Summary and Timeline, and CRS Report R41210, Medicaid and the State Children's Health Insurance Program (CHIP) Provisions in ACA: Summary and Timeline.

g. See CRS Report R41124, Medicare: Changes Made by the Reconciliation Act of 2010 to the Patient Protection and Affordable Care Act (P.L. 111-148).

h. See CRS Report R42944, Medicare, Medicaid, and Other Health Provisions in the American Taxpayer Relief Act of 2012.

i. See CRS Report R43962, The Medicare Access and CHIP Reauthorization Act of 2015 (MACRA; P.L. 114-10).

APPENDIX C. LIST OF ABBREVIATIONS

AAA	Area Agencies on Aging
ACA	Patient Protection and Affordable Care Act (P.L. 111-148, as amended)
ACF	Administration for Children and Families
ACL	Administration for Community Living

ADRC	Aging and Disability Resource Center
AHRQ	Agency for Healthcare Research and Quality
ARRA	American Recovery and Reinvestment Act of 2009 (P.L. 111-5)
ASC	Ambulatory Surgery Center
ATRA	American Taxpayer Relief Act of 2012 (P.L. 112-240)
BBA 13	Bipartisan Budget Act of 2013 (P.L. 113-67, Division A)
BBA 97	Balanced Budget Act of 1997 (P.L. 105-33)
BBA 2018	Bipartisan Budget Act of 2018
BBRA 99	Balanced Budget Refinement Act of 1999 (P.L. 106-113)
BIPA 2000	Medicare, Medicaid, and SCHIP Benefits Improvement and Protection Act of 2000 (P.L. 106-554)
CAH	Critical access hospital
CHCF	Community Health Center Fund
CHIP	State Children's Health Insurance Program
CHIPRA	Children's Health Insurance Program Reauthorization Act (P.L. 111-3)
CMS	Centers for Medicare & Medicaid Services
CPI-U	Consumer Price Index for All Urban Consumers
CRS	Congressional Research Service
CY	Calendar year
DME	Durable medical equipment
DRA	Deficit Reduction Act of 2005 (P.L. 109-171)
DSH	Disproportionate share hospital
E-FMAP	Enhanced federal medical assistance percentage
EHR	Electronic health record
FMAP	Federal medical assistance percentage
FY	Fiscal year
GAO	Government Accountability Office
GME	Graduate medical education
GPCI	Geographic Practice Cost Index
HCERA	Health Care and Education Reconciliation Act of 2010 (P.L. 111-152)
HCFAC	Health Care Fraud and Abuse Control

HH	Home health
HHS	Department of Health and Human Services
HI	Hospital Insurance
HIPAA	Health Insurance Portability and Protection Act of 1996 (P.L. 104-191)
HIT	Health information technology
HITECH	Health Information Technology for Economic and Clinical Health Act
HPOG	Health Profession Opportunity Grants
HRSA	Health Resources and Services Administration
IHS	Indian Health Service
IPPS	Medicare Inpatient Prospective Payment System
LTCH	Long-term care hospital
LTCH PPS	Long-term care hospital prospective payment system
LTSS	Long-term services and supports
MA	Medicare Advantage
MA-PD	Medicare Advantage-Prescription Drug
MACRA	Medicare Access and CHIP Reauthorization Act of 2015 (P.L. 114-10)
MAP:	Measure Applications Partnership
MCTRJCA	Middle Class Tax Relief and Job Creation Act of 2012 (P.L. 112-96)
MEDH	Medicare-dependent hospital
MedPAC	Medicare Payment Advisory Commission
MIECHV	Maternal, Infant, and Early Childhood Home Visiting
MIP	Medicare Integrity Program
MIPPA	Medicare Improvements for Patients and Providers Act of 2008 (P.L. 110-275)
MMA	Medicare Prescription Drug, Improvement, and Modernization Act of 2003 (P.L. 108- 173)
MMEA	Medicare and Medicaid Extenders Act of 2010 (P.L. 111-309)
MMSEA	Medicare, Medicaid and SCHIP Extension Act of 2007 (P.L. 110-173)

MPFS	Medicare physician fee schedule
MSA	Metropolitan Statistical Area
NHSC	National Health Service Corps
NQF	National Quality Forum
OBRA 90	Omnibus Budget Reconciliation Act of 1990 (P.L. 101-508)
OPPS:	Outpatient Prospective Payment System
PAMA	Protecting Access to Medicare Act of 2014 (P.L. 113-93)
PAMPA	Patient Access and Medicare Protection Act (P.L. 114-115)
PCORI	Patient-Centered Outcomes Research Institute
PCORTF	Patient-Centered Outcomes Research Trust Fund
PDP	Prescription Drug Plan
PHSA	Public Health Service Act
PPS	Prospective payment system
PQMP	Pediatric Quality Measures Program
PREP	Personal Responsibility Education Program
PRWORA	Personal Responsibility and Work Opportunity Reconciliation Act of 1996 (P.L. 104-193)
PSRA	Pathway for SGR Reform Act of 2013 (P.L. 113-67, Division B)
RVU	Relative value unit
SGR	Sustainable Growth Rate
SHIP	State Health Insurance Assistance Program
SMI	Supplementary Medical Insurance
SNAP	Supplemental Nutrition Assistance Program
SSA	Social Security Act
SRAE	Sexual Risk Avoidance Education
SSI	Supplemental Security Income
TAA	Trade Adjustment Assistance
TANF	State Temporary Assistance for Needy Families
TEFRA	Tax Equity and Fiscal Responsibility Act of 1982 (P.L. 97-248)
TPL	Third-party liability

TPTCCA	Temporary Payroll Tax Cut Continuation Act of 2011 (P.L. 112-78)
TRHCA	Tax Relief and Health Care Act of 2006 (P.L. 109-432)
U.S.C.	*U.S. Code*
WREA 2003	Welfare Reform Extension Act of 2003 (P.L. 108-40)
WREA 2004	Welfare Reform Extension Act of 2004 (P.L. 108-210)
WREA 2005	Welfare Reform Extension Act of 2005 (P.L. 109-4)

In: Key Congressional Reports for June 2019 ISBN: 978-1-53616-665-1
Editor: Amada A. Byrd

Chapter 4

Location of Medication-Assisted Treatment for Opioid Addiction: In Brief*

Johnathan H. Duff and Jameson A. Carter

Summary

The substantial burden of opioid abuse related to the current opioid epidemic in the United States has resulted in a disparity between the need for substance abuse treatment and the current capacity. Methadone and buprenorphine are two medications used in medication-assisted treatment (MAT) for opioid use disorder (OUD). Methadone and buprenorphine are both opioids; their use to treat opioid use disorders is often called *opioid agonist treatment* or *therapy* (OAT) or *opioid agonist MAT*. As controlled substances, methadone and buprenorphine are subject to additional regulations. Methadone may be used to treat opioid addiction within federally certified opioid treatment programs (OTP)—often referred to as methadone clinics. Buprenorphine may be used to treat opioid use disorder in two settings: (1) within an OTP and (2) outside an OTP pursuant to a Drug Addiction Treatment Act (DATA) waiver.

* This is an edited, reformatted and augmented version of Congressional Research Service Publication No. R45782, dated June 24, 2019.

The federal government has taken steps to increase the availability of MAT in response to the escalation of opioid overdoses and deaths in recent years. Policy efforts to address the opioid epidemic have corresponded with increased treatment availability, yet access to substance abuse treatment has not kept pace with the increasing rates of opioid addiction in the United States. Geographic information is important in accurately evaluating treatment capacity. Treatment location may be especially relevant to understanding the discrepancy between need and capacity. The current report identifies the geographic location of MAT providers using methadone and buprenorphine (opioid agonist treatment) in the United States. The analysis uses Substance Abuse and Mental Health Services Administration (SAMHSA) data to identify the number and location of (1) federally certified opioid treatment programs and (2) practitioners with DATA waivers. The geographic location of OTPs and DATA-waived practitioners are displayed in several national and regional maps.

Identifying the location of OAT providers may have utility in increasing accessibility to treatment. However, simply increasing capacity for treatment may not effectively increase availability (or decrease opioid-related overdoses) if treatment providers are not located in areas of need. The current analysis does not evaluate need—by locating opioid-related overdose hospital admissions and deaths for instance. It does, however, provide an initial step in assessing how treatment providers are dispersed geographically. Other factors, such as substance use treatment financing, stigma, and waiting periods for services may also affect OAT availability. Practitioners are subject to state laws and regulations regarding prescribing privileges which affect their eligibility for DATA waivers and, in turn, the availability of treatment. Congress may incorporate geographic factors in strategies designed to increase capacity and availability of treatment.

INTRODUCTION

The substantial burden of opioid abuse related to the current opioid epidemic in the United States has resulted in a disparity between the need for substance abuse treatment and the current capacity of the health care delivery system to meet that need. In 2017, over 47,600 people died of opioid-related drug overdoses in the United States.[1] In that same year, an

[1] .S. Department of Health and Human Services (HHS), National Institutes of Health (NIH), National Institute on Drug Abuse (NIDA), *Overdose Death Rates*, Updated August 2018,

estimated 11.4 million people aged 12 and older misused opioids, including 11.1 million misusers of prescription pain relievers and 886,000 heroin users.[2] The majority of individuals in need of treatment do not receive it. In 2016, one-fifth (21.1%) of those with any opioid use disorder (OUD)[3] received specialty substance abuse treatment, including 37.5% of those with heroin use disorder and 17.5% of those with prescription pain reliever use disorders.[4]

OPIOID AGONIST MEDICATION-ASSISTED TREATMENT

Medication-assisted treatment (MAT) is the combined use of medication and other services to treat addiction. MAT is widely accepted as the most effective treatment for opioid use disorder.[5] Three medications are currently used in MAT for opioid addiction: methadone, buprenorphine, and naltrexone (naloxone, a medication used to reverse opioid overdose, is not used to treat opioid use disorders).

---

https://www.drugabuse.gov/related-topics/trendsstatistics/overdose-death-rates and HHS, Centers for Disease Control and Prevention (CDC), *Opioid Overdose Deaths in the United States, 1999-2017*, NCHS Data Brief, No. 329, 2018, https://www.cdc.gov/nchs/products/databriefs/db329.htm.

[2] See HHS, SAMHSA, *Key Substance Use and Mental Health Indicators in the United States: Results from the 2017 National Survey on Drug Use and Health*, HHS Publication No. SMA 18-5068, NSDUH Series H-53, 2018, https://www.samhsa.gov/data/report/2017-nsduh-annual-national-report.

[3] *Opioid use disorder* is the official diagnostic term for "a problematic pattern of opioid use leading to clinically significant impairment or distress," as defined in the current edition of the American Psychiatric Association's Diagnostic and Statistical Manual of Mental Disorders (DSM-5).

[4] HHS, SAMHSA, *SAMHSA Shares Latest Behavioral Health Data, Including Opioid Misuse*, October 12, 2017, https://newsletter.samhsa.gov/2017/10/12/samhsa-new-data-mental-health-substance-use-including-opioids/. The data on heroin-related deaths reported in this source is drawn from HHS, Centers for Disease Control and Prevention (CDC), National Center for Health Statistics (NCHS), National Vital Statistics System (NVSS). All other data are drawn from SAMHSA's National Survey on Drug Use and Health (NSDUH).

[5] See, for example, Nora Volkow, Emily Jones, and Emily Einstein, et al., "Prevention and Treatment of Opioid Misuse and Addiction: A Review," *JAMA Psychiatry*, vol. 76, no. 2 (February 2019), pp. 208-216.

Opioid Use Disorder Treatments and Acronyms Used	
Treatment	**Description**
Buprenorphine	A synthetic opioid medication that acts as a partial agonist at opioid receptors. It does not produce the euphoria and sedation caused by full opioid agonists but is able to reduce or eliminate withdrawal symptoms and carries a low risk of overdose. It is available by prescription from qualified health providers who have obtained Drug Addiction Treatment Act of 2000 (DATA) waivers.[6]
Buprenorphine/Naloxone	Often referred to by the brand name Suboxone®, it is a combination of buprenorphine and naloxone. Naloxone is a full opioid antagonist used to block the effects of other opioids. It is activated if the buprenorphine is injected instead of dissolved by mouth.
Medication-Assisted Treatment (MAT)	The combined use of medication and other services (such as counseling) to treat addiction. Three medications are currently used in MAT for opioid addiction: methadone, buprenorphine, and naltrexone.
Methadone	A long-acting synthetic opioid agonist medication that can prevent withdrawal symptoms and reduce craving in opioid-addicted individuals. It is available through specially licensed opioid treatment programs (OTPs).
Opioid Agonist Treatment(OAT)	The use of methadone or buprenorphine in medication-assisted treatment. It is also referred to as opioid agonist MAT, opioid substitution therapy, or opioid replacement therapy.
Opioid Treatment Programs (OTPs)	Federally certified substance abuse treatment facilities—often called methadone clinics—that offer opioid medications in addition to counseling and other services for individuals addicted to heroin or other opioids.
Opioid Use Disorder (OUD)	The official diagnostic term for "a problematic pattern of opioid use leading to clinically significant impairment or distress," as defined in the current edition of the American Psychiatric Association's Diagnostic and Statistical Manual of Mental Disorders (DSM-5).
Naltrexone	The third FDA-approved medication used in MAT, it is a synthetic opioid antagonist that blocks opioids from binding to their receptors and thereby prevents any euphoric effect. Naltrexone is not an opioid and therefore is not regulated under the Controlled Substances Act.

Source: CRS analysis and also U.S. Department of Health and Human Services, National Institutes of Health, National Institute on Drug Abuse, Principles of Drug Addiction Treatment: A Research-Based Guide (Third Edition), NIH Publication No. 1 2-4 1 80, December 2012, https://www.drugabuse.gov/publications/principles-drugaddiction-treatment-research-based-guide-third-edition. Last updated January, 2018 and Suzuki, Joji, Buprenorphine Formulations: A Practical Summary for Clinicians, Psychopharmacology Institute, Clinical Psycho pharmacology Education for Prescribers CME/CE Program, September 1 1, 2017, https://psycho pharmacologyinstitute.com/substance-use-disorders/buprenorphine-formulations-practicalsummary-clinicians/.

[6] Title XXXV of P.L. 106-310.

Methadone and buprenorphine are both opioids; their use to treat opioid use disorders is often called *opioid agonist treatment* (OAT), *opioid agonist MAT*, *opioid substitution therapy*, or *opioid replacement therapy*.[7] Methadone or buprenorphine may be used both in the short term to mitigate the immediate withdrawal symptoms associated with discontinuing use of the opioid of abuse and over extended periods to maintain abstinence and prevent relapse. Descriptions of medication-assisted treatments for opioid use disorder and commonly used acronyms are included in the textbox below.

As controlled substances, methadone and buprenorphine are regulated under the Controlled Substances Act (CSA; 21 U.S.C. §§801 et seq.).[8] Under the CSA, methadone may be used to treat opioid addiction within an inpatient setting, such as a hospital, or in a federally certified opioid treatment program (OTP). Federally certified OTPs—often referred to as methadone clinics— offer opioid medications, counseling, and other services for individuals addicted to heroin or other opioids. With few exceptions, the use of methadone to treat opioid addiction is limited to OTPs. Treatment within an OTP may be in an inpatient or outpatient capacity, though typically it occurs on an outpatient basis. There are no federal limits on the number of patients that can be treated at an OTP. However, in 2016 HHS determined—through SAMHSA survey data—that an OTP could manage, on average, 262 to 334 patients at any given time.[9]

Buprenorphine may be used to treat opioid use disorder in two settings: (1) within an OTP and (2) outside an OTP pursuant to a waiver.[10] A physician or other practitioner (e.g., physician assistant or nurse

[7] In the current report, the terms *opioid agonist treatment* (OAT) or *opioid agonist MAT* will be used. An opioid "agonist" activates opioid receptors in the human brain, whereas an opioid "antagonist" blocks those same receptors from being activated.

[8] Naltrexone, which is not an opioid, does not carry an addiction risk and is not regulated under the CSA. Naltrexone may be used in an OTP, or may be provided outside an OTP by health care professionals who are allowed to prescribe drugs, without federal DATA waivers.

[9] For more details, see HHS, SAMHSA, "Medication Assisted Treatment for Opioid Use Disorders," 81 *Federal Register* 44711-44739, July 8, 2016.

[10] Federal law regulates buprenorphine differently depending on whether it is being used to treat opioid use disorders (as opposed to pain).

practitioner)[11] may obtain a waiver to administer, dispense, or prescribe buprenorphine outside an OTP. This is commonly known as a DATA waiver, drawing its name from the law that established the waiver authority: the Drug Addiction Treatment Act of 2000 (DATA 2000).[12] To qualify for a waiver, a practitioner must notify the Health and Human Services (HHS) Secretary[13] of the intent to use buprenorphine to treat opioid use disorders and must certify that he or she

- is a qualifying practitioner;[14]
- can refer patients for appropriate counseling and other services; and
- will comply with statutory limits on the number of patients that may be treated at one time.

The patient limit is 30 individuals during the first year and may increase to 100 after one year or immediately if the practitioner holds additional credentialing or operates in a qualified practice setting.[15] The patient limit may increase to 275 after one year under certain conditions specified in regulation.[16] Practitioners are subject to state laws and regulations regarding prescribing privileges and therefore may not be

---

[11] The SUPPORT Act (P.L. 115-271) expanded the definition of "qualifying other practitioner" to include clinical nurse specialists, certified registered nurse anesthetists, and certified nurse midwives. Practitioners are subject to state laws and regulations surrounding prescribing privileges and therefore may not be eligible in all states.

[12] Title XXXV of P.L. 106-310, The Children's Health Act of 2000; waivers are sometimes referred to as "X waivers."

[13] The DATA waiver system is managed by SAMHSA.

[14] The term "qualifying practitioner" is defined in 21 U.S.C. §823(g)(2)(G)(iii) to mean a qualifying physician, a qualifying other practitioner (i.e., a nurse practitioner or physician assistant), or for the period beginning on October 1, 2018 and ending on October 1, 2023, a qualifying other practitioner who is a clinical nurse specialist, certified registered nurse anesthetist, or certified nurse midwife, each of whom must meet specified requirements. Practitioners are subject to state laws and regulations regarding prescribing privileges and therefore may not be eligible in all states.

[15] 21 U.S.C. §823(g)(2)(B)(iii), as amended by the SUPPORT Act (P.L. 115-271). "Additional credentialing" is defined in 42 C.F.R. §8.2 and "qualified practice setting" is defined in 42 C.F.R. §8.615.

[16] 42 C.F.R. Part 8 Subpart F.

eligible in all states. Similar to methadone treatment, MAT with buprenorphine typically takes place in an outpatient setting.

Policy Considerations

The federal government has taken steps to increase the availability of opioid agonist MAT in response to the escalation of opioid overdoses and deaths in recent years. Both Congress and the Administration have implemented policies intended to increase access to methadone and buprenorphine, such as changes to the DATA waivers.[17] The Comprehensive Addiction and Recovery Act of 2016 (CARA; P.L. 114-198), for instance, provided qualifying nurse practitioners and physician assistants temporary eligibility to obtain DATA waivers. The SUPPORT for Patients and Communities Act (P.L. 115-271), enacted in 2018, made the authority for qualifying nurse practitioners and physician assistants to obtain DATA waivers permanent and expanded the definition of "qualifying other practitioners" to include other midlevel providers such as clinical nurse specialists, certified registered nurse anesthetists, and certified nurse midwives.[18] The law also authorized programs to establish additional comprehensive opioid recovery centers that offer a "full continuum of treatment services" including all FDA-approved medications used in MAT[19] as well as "regional centers of excellence in substance use disorder education" that would aim to improve health professional training in substance abuse treatment.[20]

---

[17] Congress has authorized and funded grant programs aimed at increasing access to treatment for opioid addiction, including but not limited to MAT. For example, Section 1003 of the 21st Century Cures Act (P.L. 114-255, enacted in December 2016) authorizes the State Targeted Response to the Opioid Crisis grant program, which supports states in addressing the opioid abuse crisis. Another example is Section 103 of the Comprehensive Addiction and Recovery Act (P.L. 114-198) which authorized funding for Community-based Coalition Enhancement Grants to Address Local Drug Crises.

[18] 42 C.F.R. §§8.610 - 8.655; of note, the term "physician" in this report refers to DATA-waived providers prior to the expanded eligibility provided by CARA. The term "practitioner" is used to include physicians and eligible midlevel providers as permitted by CARA and the SUPPORT Act.

[19] P.L. 115-271 §7121.

[20] P.L. 115-271 §7101.

Policy efforts to address the opioid epidemic have corresponded with increased MAT availability. The percentage of substance abuse treatment facilities providing buprenorphine treatment increased from 14% in 2007 to 29% of all facilities in 2017.[21] Additionally, the number of DATA-waived physicians with a 30-patient limit increased nine-fold from 2003 to 2012—from 1,800 physicians to 16,095. Physicians with a 100-patient limit tripled in the latter half of that span— from 1,937 in 2007 to 6,103 in 2012.[22]

Despite this increase, access to substance abuse treatment has not kept pace with the mounting rates of opioid addiction in the United States.[23] Additionally, while the capability to treat patients with buprenorphine has expanded through an increase in DATA waivers, practitioners with these waivers are not treating to capacity. A 2018 study by SAMHSA leadership found that the number of patients being treated by DATA-waived providers included in their study was substantially lower than the authorized waiver patient limit.[24] The percentage of clinicians prescribing buprenorphine at or near the patient limit in the month prior to the study was 13.1%.[25]

GEOGRAPHICAL ANALYSIS

Geography is essential to accurately evaluating opioid agonist MAT capacity. Treatment location may be especially relevant to understanding any discrepancy between need and capacity: where services are located may be more important than how many patients a practitioner is allowed to

[21] HHS, SAMHSA, *National Survey of Substance Abuse Treatment Services (N-SSATS): 2017. Data on Substance Abuse Treatment Facilities*, Rockville, MD, July 2018, p. 16.

[22] HHS, SAMHSA, *Medication-Assisted Treatment: Physician and Program Data*, Last updated November 26, 2018, https://www.samhsa.gov/medication-assisted-treatment/physician-program-data.

[23] Christopher Jones, Melisa Campopiano, and Grant Baldwin et al., "National and State Treatment Need and Capacity for Opioid Agonist Medication-Assisted Treatment," *American Journal of Public Health*, vol. 105, no. 8 (August 2015), pp. e55-363.

[24] Christopher M. Jones and Elinore F. McCance-Katz, "Characteristics and Prescribing Practices of Clinicians Recently Waivered to Prescribe Buprenorphine for the Treatment of Opioid Use Disorder," *Addiction*, October 15, 2018, pp. 1-12.

[25] Ibid.

treat. According to the 2018 study on DATA-waived clinicians, the top reason practitioners cited for not prescribing buprenorphine was lack of patient demand. This suggests a discrepancy between OAT practitioners and patients in need. DATA-waived practitioners may not be in the areas with the most need for treatment, for instance. Other barriers may also exist that prevent patients from accessing services. Factors affecting the treatment gap may include health insurance coverage, reimbursement for treatment services, transportation, stigma, awareness of treatment options and availability, and motivation for recovery, among others.

The current report identifies the geographic location of opioid agonist treatment providers in the United States. The analysis uses SAMHSA data to identify the number and location of (1) federally certified opioid treatment programs and (2) practitioners with DATA waivers. Data are displayed nationally as well as by county.

The location of opioid agonist MAT providers does not necessarily equate to availability of treatment. Other aforementioned factors, such as treatment costs, demand for services, wait times, and awareness of options also affect treatment availability. The current report does not attempt to evaluate the availability, accessibility, or total capacity for treatment of any area. It also does not assess need for treatment services—an essential factor in classifying discrepancies between demand for treatment and capacity of services.

Methodology

The Substance Abuse and Mental Health Services Administration, a branch of HHS which oversees the certification of opioid treatment programs and the buprenorphine waiver program, provides the number and location of OTPs and daily updates on the number and location of DATA-waived practitioners.[26] Using these data, CRS plotted 99% of OTP locations (1,652 OTPs) and 99% of publicly-available DATA-waived practitioner locations (40,016 practitioners) using the geospatial software

[26] This does not include Puerto Rico or the U.S. Territories. Not all DATA-waived practitioners are included due to some practitioners opting not to be listed publicly on SAMHSA's website.

ArcGIS.[27] As of June 1, 2019, the number of federally certified OTPs in the United States was 1,674. The total number of DATA-waived providers with a 30-patient limit exceeded 50,000 and those with a 100-patient limit exceeded 12,000.[28] The number of practitioners with a 275-patient limit totaled over 4,800.[29] This provides the capacity for at least 4 million patients to be treated with buprenorphine through DATA-waived providers.[30]

CRS generated a series of maps to depict the distribution of DATA-waived providers and neighboring OTPs in 2018. There are two maps at the national level in *Figure 1* and *Figure 2*, and two for the Northeast and parts of the Midwest in *Figure 3*. The latter maps shade in each county based on the number of DATA-waived providers in that county and demarcate each OTP with a purple dot. The shading of each county was determined using Jenks natural breaks optimization, a statistical method used to create "fair" categories. As a result, each level of shading does not follow a consistent range. The smallest shading category (1-32 DATA-waived practitioners in a county) is much smaller in range than the largest (446-871 DATA-waived practitioners in a county) on account of this method.

The Northeast region of the United States is displayed in a separate map for greater visibility of the high number of OTPs within a relatively small geographic area. (Other areas experiencing highly clustered OTPs, such as California and Florida, are more easily discerned on the national map and are therefore not displayed in additional maps.) Parts of the Midwest are displayed in a regional map for greater visibility of areas

---

[27] http://www.arcgis.com/index.html.

[28] As aforementioned, the current geospatial analysis did not include all DATA-waived practitioners due to some practitioners opting not to be listed publicly on SAMHSA's website.

[29] HHS, SAMHSA, *Medication-Assisted Treatment: Physician and Program Data*, Last updated November 26, 2018, https://www.samhsa.gov/medication-assisted-treatment/physician-program-data.

[30] Ibid. Since there are no federal limits on the number of patients that can be treated at an OTP, the buprenorphine treatment capacity analysis here does not include patients who could be treated with buprenorphine at an OTP.

disproportionately affected by the opioid crisis.[31] These maps present location of OAT providers only. Geography is one indication of adequacy of treatment capacity but other factors—such as population density and the size of the affected populations in the area—are also relevant. This analysis only examines the geographic location of OAT providers.

Results

Results depicted in *Figure 1*, *Figure 2*, and *Figure 3* show that opioid agonist medication-assisted treatment services are not evenly distributed across the country.[32] The maps in *Figure 2* and *Figure 3* depict the location of federally certified OTPs and the number of DATA-waived practitioners in each county. Results from this analysis indicated that:

- 1,217 counties (39% of counties nationally)—populated by an estimated 17.5 million people (of 321 million nationally, or 5.5% of the population)—had no DATA-waived practitioners.
- Nearly 2,500 counties (80% nationally), populated by an estimated 77.5 million people (24% of the population), had no OTPs and 1,202 counties (38%), populated by 16.8 million people (5.2%), had neither an OTP nor a DATA-waived practitioner.
- Of the over 1,200 counties with no OAT providers, nearly half (45%) are classified as rural according to the U.S. Census.[33] These counties are primarily located in the Midwest and South; Texas

---

[31] Defined here as Ohio, West Virginia, Kentucky, Indiana, western Pennsylvania, and eastern Illinois.

[32] Further, OTPs are not necessarily accessible to all residents in a given area. For instance, several states/localities operate OTPs through correctional facilities. The Bernalillo County Detention Center in New Mexico, for example, operates an OTP for inmates, as does Riker's Island in New York. Generally, states have not equipped their correctional facilities with OTPs (with the exception of Rhode Island which administers a system of OTPs through its correctional facilities). Arizona, Connecticut, DC, Georgia, Maryland, New York, and Rhode Island all have OTPs located in, or affiliated with, correctional facilities. CRS was not able to determine whether the population served is strictly inmates however. In all, CRS was able to identify 13 OTPs servicing detention centers in these data. Therefore, the presence of an OTP may not indicate that OTP is accessible for the general population in some cases.

[33] Defined as having no urban cluster or urbanized area within its boundaries. Urban clusters are defined as having a population of 2,500-50,000 people and urbanized areas are defined as having 50,000 or more people.

(13% of counties with no OTPs or DATA-waived practitioners), Georgia (6%), Kansas (6%), Nebraska (5%), Iowa (5%), and Missouri (5%) have the highest percentages of counties with no OTPs or DATA-waived providers.
- Twenty-five counties with no OTPs or DATA-waived practitioners had more than 50,000 residents.[34]

It is important to consider that county size and population are not necessarily indicators of substance abuse treatment need. Counties are also not equivalent in geographic area, shape, and population size and therefore comparisons on treatment availability strictly across the county level may not be appropriate. Additionally, the absence of OAT providers does not necessarily equate to lack of access (adjacent counties may offer treatment for instance and patients may travel for inpatient treatment). Similarly, the presence of providers does not necessarily equate to treatment availability, particularly within counties that encompass large geographic areas.

Policy Implications

Federal lawmakers have sought to increase the capacity for opioid use disorder treatment with MAT to address the ongoing opioid epidemic. Thus far in the 116th Congress, policymakers have introduced nearly a dozen bills explicitly pertaining to opioid use disorder treatment expansion. For example, one bill would remove some requirements for health providers to receive DATA waivers to administer buprenorphine, with the intention that more practitioners would then pursue these waivers.

Identifying the location of OAT providers may be essential to increasing accessibility to treatment. Simply increasing capacity for treatment may not effectively increase availability (or decrease opioid-related overdoses) if treatment providers are not located in areas of need. While the current analysis does not evaluate need—by locating opioid-

[34] Livingston Parish in Louisiana (137,096 people), Kendall County in Illinois (122,933), Carver County in Minnesota (98,799), Platte County in Missouri (96,899), and Vermillion County in Illinois (79,207) had the highest number of residents of the counties with no OTPs or DATA-waived providers.

related overdose hospital admissions and deaths for instance—it does provide an initial step in assessing how treatment providers are dispersed geographically.[35] Other factors, such as substance use treatment financing, may also affect OAT availability. Practitioners are also subject to state laws and regulations regarding prescribing privileges which affect the eligibility of providers for DATA waivers and, in turn, the availability of treatment.

Congress may consider incorporating geographic factors in strategies designed to increase capacity and availability of treatment. For instance, policymakers may acknowledge the dispersion of treatment providers within small geographic units and the proximity of OTPs to DATA-waived practitioners when drafting legislation. Rural areas may not have the same volume of need for substance use disorder treatment as urban areas, yet they may possess additional barriers to care that make accessibility to treatment challenging. For example, patients traveling long distances to receive daily methadone at an OTP may face obstacles related to transportation or infrastructure that make continuity of treatment difficult. Additionally, DATA-waived providers alone may not have the resources to provide complementary services such as counseling and behavioral therapies, or housing and vocational services.

Some individual states have sought to address geographical obstacles to care through treatment and policy strategies. Vermont, for example, operates a "hub-and-spoke" system, in which patients seeking treatment for OUD establish care at an OTP (the "hub") where they receive more intensive services, often during their initial entry to treatment when such concentration of services is more necessary.[36] Once patients are stabilized, they transition to a DATA-waived provider in their community for maintenance treatment with buprenorphine (the "spoke"), and other services. If patients relapse, they may return to the OTP until they are

[35] Indicators of treatment need, such as drug overdose death and hospital admission data, are not available for every county. Therefore, CRS was not able to compare treatment capacity with need for treatment on a national scale.

[36] John R. Brooklyn and Stacey C. Sigmon, "Vermont Hub-and-Spoke Model of Care for Opioid Use Disorder: Development, Implementation, and Impact," *Journal of Addiction Medicine*, vol. 11, no. 4 (2017), pp. 286-292.

ready to transition back to outpatient buprenorphine, and the cycle continues. Throughout their treatment, patients are followed by the same care management team who assist them in finding and accessing appropriate services. Vermont officials sought to ensure OTPs were distributed throughout the state (see *Figure 3*). A part of Vermont's hub and spoke strategy has been to divide resources geographically throughout the state to reduce the number of areas without treatment. Other states, such as New Jersey and Washington, addressed geographic barriers by operating mobile methadone units, known as "methadone vans," which travelled from OTPs to provide daily methadone medication to rural and other hard-to-reach patients.[37] Other states have offered similar mobile services with buprenorphine.

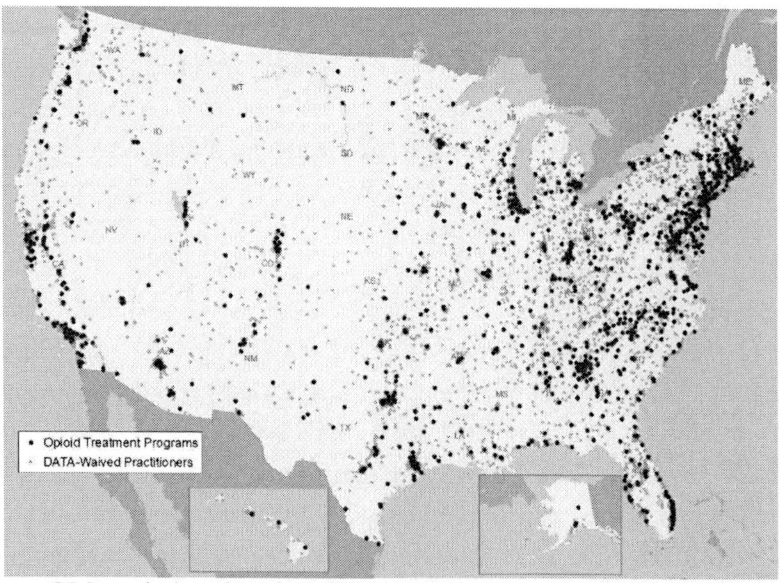

Source: CRS analysis using data from the Substance Abuse and Mental Health Services Administration as of May 9, 2019.

Figure 1. Location of Opioid Treatment Programs and DATA-Waived Practitioners in the United States.

[37] See, for example, Gerod Hall, Charles J. Neighbors, and Jude Iheoma, et al., "Mobile opioid agonist treatment and public funding expands treatment for disenfranchised opioid-dependent individuals," *Journal of Substance Abuse Treatment*, vol. 46 (2014), pp. 511-515.

Increasing the quantity of treatment providers may only be effective in addressing the opioid epidemic if access to treatment is also addressed. Both examples provided above, for instance, seek to not only expand treatment capacity, but also enhance accessibility by attending to location of services in relation to the patient population. Geography alone is not the only barrier; stigma, financing, and patient willingness may also influence the amount and utilization of services. Congress may explore additional solutions, such as the use of telemedicine services where possible. Nevertheless, identifying the location of providers may be an important step for policymakers seeking to increase availability of treatment for opioid use disorder.

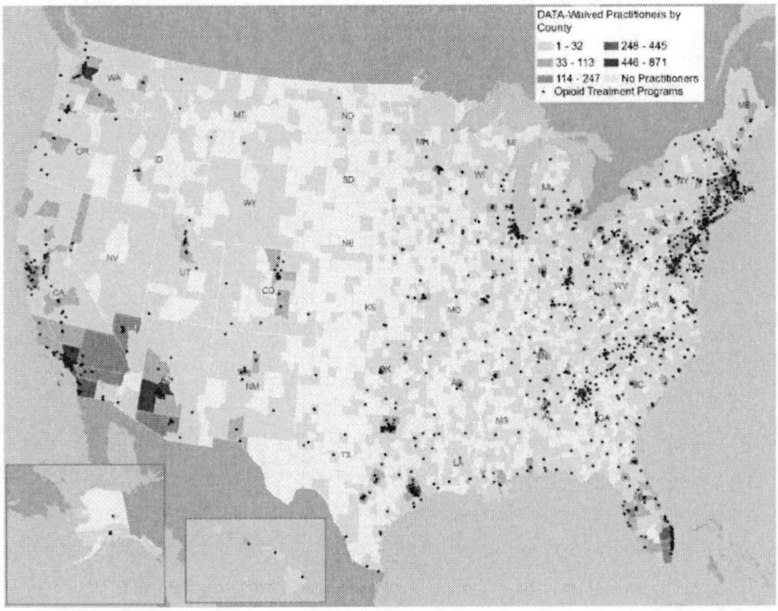

Source: CRS analysis using data from the Substance Abuse and Mental Health Services Administration as of May 9, 2019.

Figure 2. Location of Opioid Treatment Programs and DATA-Waived Practitioners by County in the United States.

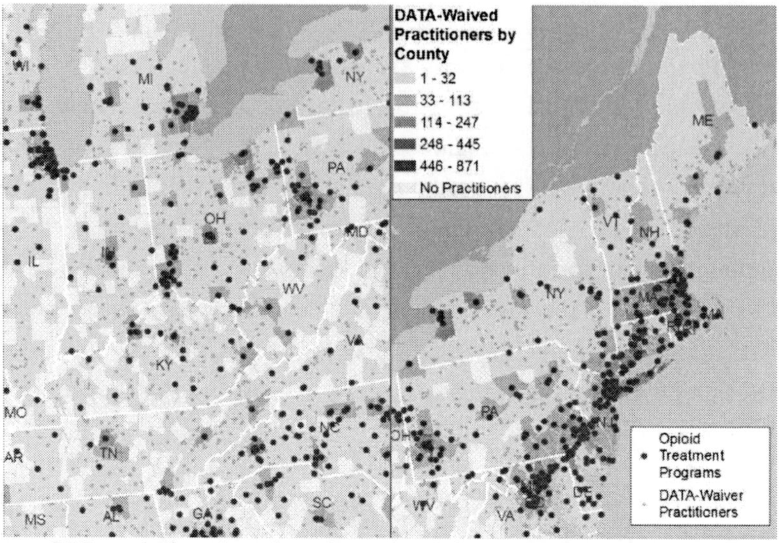

Source: CRS analysis using data from the Substance Abuse and Mental Health Services Administration as of May 9. 2019.

Notes: States in the Northeast region are displayed for greater visibility of the high number of OTPs within a relatively small geographic area. Parts of the Midwest, including Ohio, West Virginia, Kentucky, Indiana, western Pennsylvania, and eastern Illinois are displayed for greater visibility of areas disproportionately affected by the opioid crisis.

Figure 3. Location of Opioid Treatment Programs and DATA-Waived Practitioners by County in Selected Regions.

In: Key Congressional Reports for June 2019 ISBN: 978-1-53616-665-1
Editor: Amada A. Byrd

Chapter 5

THE OPIOID EPIDEMIC: SUPPLY CONTROL AND CRIMINAL JUSTICE POLICY - FREQUENTLY ASKED QUESTIONS*

Lisa N. Sacco, Kristin Finklea, Susan V. Lawrence, Liana W. Rosen and Clare Ribando Seelke

SUMMARY

Over the last several years, lawmakers in the United States have responded to rising drug overdose deaths, which increased four-fold from 1999 to 2017, with a variety of legislation, hearings, and oversight activities. In 2017, more than 70,000 people died from drug overdoses, and approximately 68% of those deaths involved an opioid.

Many federal agencies are involved in domestic and foreign efforts to combat opioid abuse and the continuing increase in opioid related overdose deaths. A subset of those agencies confront the supply side (some may also confront the demand side) of the opioid epidemic. The primary federal agency involved in drug enforcement, including

---

* This is an edited, reformatted and augmented version of a Congressional Research Service publication R45790, prepared for Members and Committees of Congress dated June 28, 2019.

prescription opioids diversion control, is the Drug Enforcement Administration (DEA). Other federal agencies that address the illicit opioid supply include, but are not limited to, the Federal Bureau of Investigation, Offices of the U.S. Attorneys, Office of Justice Programs, U.S. Customs and Border Protection, U.S. Department of State, U.S. Postal Inspection Service, and Office of National Drug Control Policy. This chapter focuses on efforts from these departments and agencies only.

Lawmakers have addressed opioid abuse as both a public health and a criminal justice issue, and Congress enacted several new laws in the 114th and 115th Congresses. These include the Comprehensive Addiction and Recovery Act of 2016 (CARA; P.L. 114-198), the 21st Century Cures Act (Cures Act; P.L. 114-255), and most recently the SUPPORT for Patients and Communities Act (SUPPORT Act; P.L. 115-271). Congress also provided funds specifically to address the opioid epidemic in FY2017-FY2019 appropriations.

This chapter answers common supply and criminal justice-related questions that have arisen as drug overdose deaths in the United States continue to increase. It does *not* provide a comprehensive overview of opioid abuse as a criminal justice issue. The report is divided into the following sections:

- Overview of the Opioid Epidemic in the United States;
- Overview of the Opioid Supply;
- Opioids and Domestic Supply Control Policy;
- Opioids and Foreign Supply Control Policy;
- Recent Congressional Action on the Opioid Epidemic; and
- The Opioid Epidemic and State Criminal Justice Policies.

Over the last several years, the public and lawmakers in the United States have been alarmed over the increasing number of drug overdose deaths, most of which have involved opioids. Congress has responded to the issue through legislative activity, oversight, and funding, while the Administration has sought to reduce the supply and demand of illicit drugs through enforcement, prevention, and treatment.

This FAQ report answers questions about the opioid epidemic and federal efforts to control the supply of opioids. It does not provide a comprehensive overview of opioid abuse and the criminal justice response. Instead, it answers common questions that have arisen due to rising drug overdose deaths and the availability of illicit opioids in the United States.

OVERVIEW OF THE OPIOID EPIDEMIC IN THE UNITED STATES

This section answers questions on the nature of the opioid epidemic in the United States. The answers provide background on the types of opioids that are being abused, the associated harm to the abusers of these substances, and the extent of the abuse.

What is an Opioid?

Terminology: Opioids and Opiates

In current usage, the term "opioids" refers to all drugs derived from the opium poppy or emulating the effects of opium-derived drugs. Technically, the term "opiates" refers to natural compounds found in the opium poppy, and "opioids" refers to synthetic compounds that emulate the effects of opiates. In either case, the drugs act on opioid receptors in the brain. This chapter relies on current usage of the term opioids, to include both natural and synthetic opioids.

An opioid is a type of drug that, when ingested, binds to opioid receptors in the body—many of which control a person's pain[1]. While opioids are medically used to alleviate pain, some are abused by being used in a way other than prescribed (e.g., in greater quantity) or taken without a doctor's prescription.[2] Many prescription pain medications, such

[1] U.S. Department of Health and Human Services (HHS), Centers for Disease Control and Prevention (CDC), "Opioid Basics—Commonly Used Terms," https://www.cdc.gov/drugoverdose/opioids/terms.html.

[2] U.S. Department of Health and Human Services (HHS), National Institutes of Health (NIH), National Institute on Drug Abuse (NIDA), *Opioids*, June 2018, https://www.drugabuse.gov/drugs-abuse/opioids. This CRS report uses the common term "abuse" to encompass a range of behaviors that are not limited to addiction. Such behaviors are variously described as "illicit use," "non-medical use," or "misuse," among other terms. See, for example, the terms used in American College of Preventive Medicine, *Use, Abuse, Misuse & Disposal of Prescription Pain Medication: Clinical Reference*, Washington, DC, 2011; and Federation of State Medical Boards, *Model Policy on the Use of Opioid Analgesics in the Treatment of Chronic Pain*, July 2013, pp. 15-18.

as hydrocodone and fentanyl, are opioids, as are some illicit drugs, such as heroin.

How many Americans Abuse Opioids?

In its annual National Survey on Drug Use and Health (NSDUH), the Substance Abuse and Mental Health Services Administration (SAMHSA) does not ask questions about "opioids" specifically; rather, it asks respondents about their use of heroin and misuse of prescription pain relievers in two separate questions.[3] In 2017, SAMHSA estimated that 11.4 million people misused an opioid at least once in the past year—this includes 11.1 million prescription pain reliever "misusers"[4] and 886,000 heroin users.[5]

In 2017, SAMHSA also estimated that 3.2 million Americans ages 12 and older (1.2% of the population 12 and older) were current "misusers" of prescription pain relievers, and approximately 494,000 Americans ages 12 and older (0.2% of the population 12 and older) were current users[6] of heroin.[7]

---

[3] Subtypes of pain relievers include hydrocodone, oxycodone, tramadol, codeine, morphine, fentanyl, buprenorphine, oxymorphone, Demerol®, hydromorphone, and methadone. See U.S. Department of Health and Human Services (HHS), Substance Abuse and Mental Health Services Administration (SAMHSA), *Results from the 2017 National Survey on Drug Use and Health: Detailed Tables*, September 2018, Table 1.1A (hereinafter, *Results from the 2017 National Survey on Drug Use and Health: Detailed Tables*) and *Methodological Summary and Definitions*, Table C-1, https://www.samhsa.gov/data/.

[4] SAMHSA defines "misuse" of prescription drugs as "use in any way not directed by a doctor including use without a prescription of one's own medication; use in greater amounts, more often, or longer than told to take a drug; or use in any other way not directed by a doctor." Prescription drugs do not include over-the-counter drugs.

[5] Some respondents fell into both categories, which is why the total (11.4 million) is lower than the two categories combined; U.S. Department of Health and Human Services (HHS), Substance Abuse and Mental Health Services Administration (SAMHSA), *Key substance use and mental health indicators in the United States: Results from the 2017 National Survey on Drug Use and Health,* 2018, https://www.samhsa.gov/data/.

[6] SAMHSA defines "current use" as having used at least once in the past month.

[7] *Results from the 2017 National Survey on Drug Use and Health: Detailed Tables.*

The University of Michigan administers an annual Monitoring the Future Survey[8], which measures drug use behaviors among 8th, 10th, and 12th graders; college students; and young adults. In 2018, 3.4% of surveyed 12th graders[9] were current users of "narcotics other than heroin", and 0.1% of surveyed 8th, 10th, and 12th graders were current users of heroin.[10]

What is the Physical Harm Associated with Opioid Abuse?

For chronic and severe pain, opioids can improve the functioning of legitimate pain patients; however, there are short- and long-term physical risks of abusing opioids. For example, nonfatal overdoses have been associated with a number of health issues, including brain injury, pulmonary and respiratory problems, hypothermia, kidney and liver failure, seizures, and others.[11] The most severe physical harm associated with opioid abuse is death due to overdose. Drug overdose deaths have increased four-fold from 16,849 in 1999 to 70,237 in 2017. Of the 70,237 overdose deaths, 47,600 (67.8%) involved opioids.[12] The main driver of drug overdose deaths overall is synthetic opioids.[13] Reports indicate that

---

[8] Monitoring the Future is funded by the National Institute of Drug Abuse, a component of the National Institutes of Health.

[9] 8th and 10th graders were not reported because the authors considered the data for this question from 8th and 10th graders to be of questionable validity.

[10] Only drug use not under a doctor's orders is included. A list of example narcotics, including Vicodin, OxyContin, and Percocet, was provided to the respondents. For more information, see Lloyd D. Johnston, et al., *Monitoring the Future, National Survey Results on Drug Use: 2018 Overview, Key Findings on Adolescent Drug Use*, The University of Michigan Institute for Social Research, January 2019, Table 7, *Trends in 30-Day Prevalence of Use of Various Drugs for Grades 8, 10, and 12 Combined.*

[11] Kathryn F. Hawk, Federico E. Vaca, and Gail D'Onofrio, "Reducing Fatal Opioid Overdose: Prevention, Treatment and Harm Reduction Strategies," *Yale Journal of Biology and Medicine*, vol. 88, no. 3 (September 3, 2015), pp. 235-245.

[12] U.S. Department of Health and Human Services (HHS), Centers for Disease Control and Prevention (CDC), *Drug Overdose Deaths* and *Understanding the Epidemic*, https://www.cdc.gov/drugoverdose/index.html; CDC, *Drug and Opioid-Involved Overdose Deaths—United States, 2013–2017*, Morbidity and Mortality Weekly Report (MMWR), January 4, 2019; and CDC, *Data Brief 294. Drug Overdose Deaths in the United States, 1999-2016*, data table for Figure 1, "Age-adjusted drug overdose death rates: United States, 1999-2016."

[13] The synthetic opioid category includes synthetic drugs such as fentanyl and tramadol, but methadone is excluded because the CDC tracks methadone deaths separately. See U.S.

recent increases in overdose deaths are most likely driven by illicitly manufactured fentanyl.[14]

Aside from the harm associated with fatal and nonfatal opioid overdoses, addiction is a primary harm associated with opioids. Licit and illicit opioids are highly addictive.[15] Addiction and general misuse of opioids have contributed to a series of public health, welfare, and social problems that have been widely discussed in public forums.[16]

Which States are Experiencing a High Number and/or Rate of Overdose Deaths?

The numbers and rates of drug overdose deaths vary by state and region of the United States. Table 1 shows the number of deaths and age-adjusted overdose death rates[17] for each state and the national totals for 2017. As illustrated in Figure 1, the states east of the Mississippi River have comparatively higher rates of drug overdose deaths than states west of the Mississippi River, although New Mexico, Arizona, and Utah all rank in the top half of states for age-adjusted rates of drug overdose deaths.

Department of Health and Human Services (HHS), Centers for Disease Control and Prevention (CDC), *Drug Overdose Deaths*, https://www.cdc.gov/drugoverdose/data/statedeaths.html.

[14] U.S. Department of Health and Human Services (HHS), Centers for Disease Control and Prevention (CDC), *Drug and Opioid-Involved Overdose Deaths – United States, 2013-2017*, Morbidity and Mortality Weekly Report, January 4, 2019, https://www.cdc.gov/mmwr/volumes/67/wr/mm675152e1.htm.

[15] Nora D. Volkow, *What Science Tells Us About Opioid Abuse and Addiction*, National Institute on Drug Abuse, Testimony before the Senate Judiciary Committee, January 27, 2016, https://www.drugabuse.gov/about-nida/legislative-activities/testimony-to-congress/2016/what-science-tells-us-about-opioid-abuse-addiction.

[16] Ibid.; Centers for Disease Control and Prevention, *2018 Annual Surveillance Report of Drug-Related Risks and Outcomes–United States*, Surveillance Special Report., August 31, 2018, https://www.cdc.gov/drugoverdose/pdf/pubs/2018-cdc-drug-surveillance-report.pdf; and National Institute on Drug Abuse, *Opioid Overdose Crisis*, revised January 2019, https://www.drugabuse.gov/drugs-abuse/opioids/opioid-overdose-crisis.

[17] [17] CDC calculated age-adjusted death rates as deaths per 100,000 in population using the direct method and the 2000 standard U.S. population. Crude death rates are influenced by the age distribution of a state's population. Age-adjusting the rates ensures that differences from one year to another or between two areas are not due to differences in the age distribution of a state's population.

Table 1. Total Numbers and Age-Adjusted Rates of Drug Overdose Deaths, 2017

Ranked from highest to lowest age-adjusted rate of drug overdose deaths			
State	**Deaths**	**Population**	**Age-Adjusted Rate per 100,000**
West Virginia	974	1,815,857	57.8
Ohio	5,111	11,658,609	46.3
Pennsylvania	5,388	12,805,537	44.3
District of Columbia	310	693,972	44.0
Kentucky	1,566	4,454,189	37.2
Delaware	338	961,939	37.0
New Hampshire	467	1,342,795	37.0
Maryland	2,247	6,052,177	36.3
Maine	424	1,335,907	34.4
Massachusetts	2,168	6,859,819	31.8
Rhode Island	320	1,059,639	31.0
Connecticut	1,072	3,588,184	30.9
New Jersey	2,685	9,005,644	30.0
Indiana	1,852	6,666,818	29.4
Michigan	2,694	9,962,311	27.8
Tennessee	1,776	6,715,984	26.6
Florida	5,088	20,984,400	25.1
New Mexico	493	2,088,070	24.8
Louisiana	1,108	4,684,333	24.5
North Carolina	2,414	10,273,419	24.1
Missouri	1,367	6,113,532	23.4
Vermont	134	623,657	23.2
Utah	650	3,101,833	22.3
Arizona	1,532	7,016,270	22.2
United States	70,237	325,719,178	21.7
Illinois	2,778	12,802,023	21.6
Nevada	676	2,998,039	21.6
Wisconsin	1,177	5,795,483	21.2
South Carolina	1,008	5,024,369	20.5
Alaska	147	739,795	20.2
Oklahoma	775	3,930,864	20.1
New York	3,921	19,849,399	19.4
Alabama	835	4,874,747	18.0
Virginia	1,507	8,470,020	17.9
Colorado	1,015	5,607,154	17.6
Arkansas	446	3,004,279	15.5
Washington	1,169	7,405,743	15.2
Georgia	1,537	10,429,379	14.7
Idaho	236	1,716,943	14.4
Hawaii	203	1,427,538	13.8

Table 1. (Continued)

Ranked from highest to lowest age-adjusted rate of drug overdose deaths			
State	**Deaths**	**Population**	**Age-Adjusted Rate per 100,000**
Minnesota	733	5,576,606	13.3
Oregon	530	4,142,776	12.4
Mississippi	354	2,984,100	12.2
Wyoming	69	579,315	12.2
Kansas	333	2,913,123	11.8
California	4,868	39,536,653	11.7
Montana	119	1,050,493	11.7
Iowa	341	3,145,711	11.5
Texas	2,989	28,304,596	10.5
North Dakota	68	755,393	9.2
South Dakota	73	869,666	8.5
Nebraska	152	1,920,076	8.1

Source: CRS presentation of data from U.S. Department of Health and Human Services (HHS), Centers for Disease Control and Prevention (CDC), National Center for Health Statistics (NCHS), NCHS-Drug Poisoning Mortality by State: United States, 2016, https://data.cdc.gov/NCHS/NCHS-Drug-Poisoning-Mortality-by-State- United-Stat/xbxb-epbu. Population estimates are from U.S. Census Bureau, American Fact Finder, Annual Estimates of the Resident Population: April 1, 2010, to July 1, 2017, *2017 Population Estimates*.

Note: CDC calculated age-adjusted death rates as deaths per 100,000 in population using the direct method and the 2000 standard U.S. population. Crude death rates are influenced by the age distribution of a state's population. Age-adjusting the rates ensures that differences from one year to another or between two areas are not due to differences in the age distribution of a state's population.

The Drug Enforcement Administration (DEA) and the Centers for Disease Control and Prevention (CDC) have indicated that overdose deaths have increased in states also reporting large increases in fentanyl seizures.[18] In addition, there is reportedly a "strong relationship" between the number of synthetic opioid deaths and the number of fentanyl reports in the National Forensic Laboratory Information System (NFLIS).[19] The National Institute on Drug Abuse (NIDA) reports that the number of

[18] U.S. Department of Health and Human Services (HHS), Centers for Disease Control and Prevention (CDC), *Increases in Fentanyl Drug Confiscations and Fentanyl-related Overdose Fatalities*, October 26, 2015, https://emergency.cdc.gov/han/han00384.asp; and U.S. Drug Enforcement Administration (DEA), *2018 National Drug Threat Assessment*, October 2018, p. 27 (hereinafter, *2018 National Drug Threat Assessment*).

[19] The DEA manages the NFLIS, which is a program that systematically collects drug chemistry analysis results from federal, state, and local forensic laboratories.

fentanyl-related deaths is likely underestimated because some medical examiners do not test for fentanyl and some death certificates do not list specific drugs.[20]

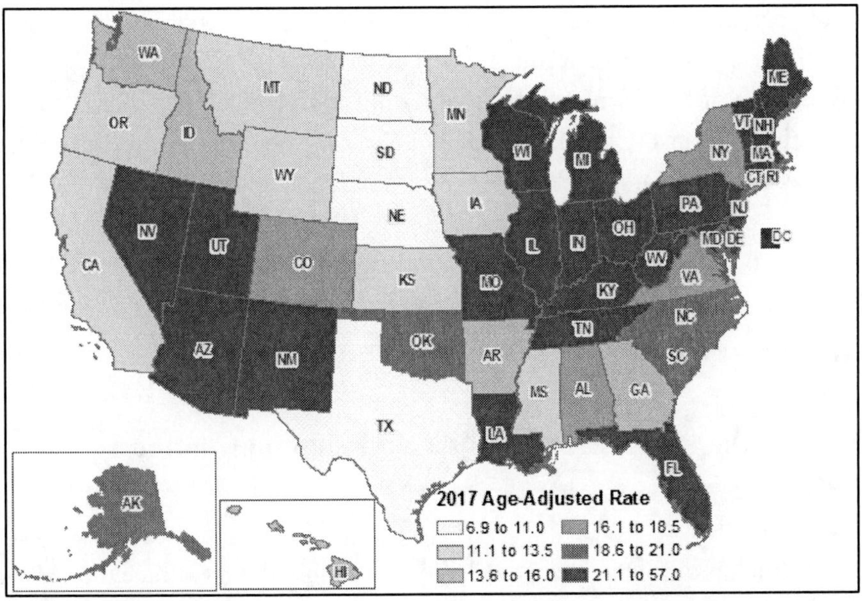

Source: CRS presentation of data from U.S. Department of Health and Human Services (HHS), Centers for Disease Control and Prevention (CDC), Drug Overdose Death Data, 2017, https://www.cdc.gov/drugoverdose/ data/ statedeaths.html.

Notes: CDC calculated age-adjusted death rates as deaths per 100,000 in population using the direct method and the 2000 standard U.S. population. Crude death rates are influenced by the age distribution of a state's population. Age-adjusting the rates ensures that differences from one year to another or between two areas are not due to differences in the age distribution of the states' populations.

Figure 1. Age-Adjusted Rates of Drug Overdose Deaths, 2017.

---

[20] U.S. Department of Health and Human Services (HHS), National Institutes of Health (NIH), National Institute on Drug Abuse (NIDA), *Addressing America's Fentanyl Crisis*, April 6, 2017, https://www.drugabuse.gov/about-nida/ noras-blog/2017/04/addressing-americas-fentanyl-crisis.

OVERVIEW OF THE OPIOID SUPPLY

Heroin, fentanyl, and prescription opioids are significant drug threats in the United States—in 2017, approximately 44% of domestic local law enforcement agencies responding[21] to the National Drug Threat Survey (NDTS) reported heroin as the greatest drug threat in their area.[22] While the percentage of NDTS respondents reporting high availability of controlled prescription drugs (CPDs),[23] which include some opioids, has declined over the last several years (75% of NDTS respondents reported high availability in 2014, compared to 52% in 2017), the reported availability of heroin has increased (30% reported high availability in 2014, compared to 49% in 2017).[24] Further, there has been a rise in the availability of illicit fentanyl—the primary synthetic opioid available in the United States.[25]

What is the Recent History of the Opioid Supply in the United States?

While opioids have been available in the United States since the 1800s, the market for these drugs shifted significantly beginning in the 1990s. This section focuses on this latter period (see Figure 2).

Prescription Opioid Supply

In the 1990s, the availability and abuse of prescription opioids, such as hydrocodone and oxycodone, increased as the legitimate production,[26] and

---

[21] For the 2017 NDTS, the DEA received 5,155 responses from 10,650 law enforcement agencies surveyed across the country. The DEA did not conduct the NDTS in 2018.

[22] U.S. Drug Enforcement Administration (DEA), *2017 National Drug Threat Assessment*, November 2017.

[23] Not all controlled prescription drugs (CPDs) are opioids. According to the DEA, CPDs include, but are not limited to, "narcotics (e.g., Vicodin, OxyContin), depressants (e.g., Valium, Xanax), stimulants (e.g., Adderall, Ritalin), and anabolic steroids (e.g., Anadrol, Oxandrin)." See U.S. Drug Enforcement Administration (DEA), *2017 National Drug Threat Assessment*, November 2017, p. 25.

[24] Ibid.; U.S. Drug Enforcement Administration (DEA), *2015 National Drug Threat Assessment Summary*, October 2015, p. 125; and *2018 National Drug Threat Assessment*, p. vi.

[25] *2018 National Drug Threat Assessment*, p. 22.

[26] According to the CDC, in the 1990s healthcare providers began using opioids "to treat chronic pain (not related to cancer), such as arthritis and back pain. As this continued, more opioid

the subsequent diversion of some of these drugs, increased sharply.[27] This continued into the early 2000s, as illegitimate prescription opioid users turned to family and friends, "doctor shopping," bad-acting physicians,[28] pill mills,[29] the internet, pharmaceutical theft, and prescription fraud to obtain prescription opioids.

The federal government has used varied approaches to reduce the unlawful prescription drug supply and prescription drug abuse, including diversion control through grants for state prescription drug monitoring programs[30]; a crackdown on pill mills; increased regulation of internet pharmacies[31]; the reformulation of a commonly abused prescription opioid, OxyContin® (oxycodone hydrochloride controlled-release)[32]; and the rescheduling of hydrocodone.[33]

Some experts have highlighted a connection between the crackdown on the unlawful supply of prescription drugs and the subsequent rise in the availability and abuse of heroin (discussed in the next section). Heroin is a cheaper alternative to prescription opioids, and may be accessible to some

---

prescriptions were written, for more days per prescription, in higher doses." See CDC, *Vital Signs – Opioid Prescribing*, https://www.cdc.gov/vitalsigns/opioids/ index.html.

[27] U.S. Department of Justice, National Drug Intelligence Center, *National Drug Threat Assessment 2005*, February 2005.

[28] One such doctor was David Procter, who established a pill mill operation from 1992 through 2001 in South Shore, KY. He is viewed as the "godfather of pills." See, for example, NPR, "How Heroin Made its Way From Rural Mexico to Small-Town America," May 19, 2015.

[29] "Pill mill" is a term used to describe a doctor, clinic, or pharmacy that is prescribing or dispensing narcotics inappropriately or for nonmedical reasons. They may be disguised as independent pain-management centers. They tend to open and shut down quickly to evade law enforcement.

[30] For more information on prescription drug monitoring programs, see CRS Report R42593, *Prescription Drug Monitoring Programs*.

[31] In response to the problem of rogue internet websites that illegally sell and dispense controlled prescription drugs, Congress passed the Ryan Haight Online Pharmacy Consumer Protection Act of 2008 (P.L. 110-425), which amended the Controlled Substances Act to expressly regulate online pharmacies. For more information, see CRS Report R43559, *Prescription Drug Abuse*.

[32] FDA approved the reformulation of OxyContin® to make it harder to crush and abuse. FDA also required a label warning of its addictive quality.

[33] On August 22, 2014, the DEA published a final rule in the *Federal Register* that administratively reschedules hydrocodone combination products from Schedule III to Schedule II, which subjects anyone who manufactures, distributes, or dispenses hydrocodone combination products to the more stringent regulatory requirements and administrative, civil, and criminal sanctions that are applicable to Schedule II controlled substances. For more information on these actions, see CRS Report R43559, *Prescription Drug Abuse*.

who are seeking an opioid high. Notably, while most users of prescription drugs will not go on to use heroin, accessibility and price are central factors cited by patients with opioid dependence who decide to turn to heroin.[34]

In October 2018, the Substance Use-Disorder Prevention that Promotes Opioid Recovery and Treatment for Patients and Communities Act (SUPPORT Act; P.L. 115-271) imposed tighter oversight of opioid production and distribution, required additional reporting and safeguards to address fraud, and limited Medicare coverage of prescription opioids.[35] Also in 2018, the DEA proposed a "significant" reduction in opioid manufacturing for 2019.[36] In its final order setting the aggregate production quota for certain controlled substances in 2019, the DEA noted that it "has observed a decline in the number of prescriptions written for schedule II opioids since 2014 and will continue to set aggregate production quotas to meet the medical needs of the United States while combating the opioid crisis."[37]

---

[34] William N. Evans, Ethan M.J. Lieber, and Patrick Power, "How the Reformulation of Oxycontin Ignited the Heroin Epidemic," *The Review of Economics and Statistics*, vol. CI, no. 1 (March 2019); U.S. Department of Health and Human Services (HHS), National Institutes of Health (NIH), National Institute on Drug Abuse (NIDA), *Prescription Drugs and Heroin*, December 2015; Pradip K. Muhuri, Joseph C. Gfroerer, and M. Christine Davies, *Associations of Nonmedical Pain Reliever Use and Initiation of Heroin Use in the United States*, U.S. Department of Health and Human Services (HHS), Substance Abuse and Mental Health Services Administration (SAMHSA), Center for Behavioral Health Statistics and Quality, August 2013, http://www.samhsa.gov/data/2k13/DataReview/DR006/ nonmedical-pain-reliever-use-2013.pdf; Theodore J. Cicero, Matthew S. Ellis, and Hilary L. Surratt, "Effect of Abuse- Deterrent Formulation of Oxycontin," *New England Journal of Medicine*, vol. 367, no. 2 (July 12, 2012), pp. 187-189; U.S. Department of Justice (DOJ), National Drug Intelligence Center (NDIC), *National Drug Threat Assessment 2011*, August 2011, p. 37; and DOJ, NDIC, *National Drug Threat Assessment 2003*, "Narcotics", January 2003.

[35] See CRS Report R45449, *The SUPPORT for Patients and Communities Act (P.L.115-271): Medicare Provisions*; CRS Report R45423, *Public Health and Other Related Provisions in P.L 115-271, the SUPPORT for Patients and Communities Act*; and CRS Report R45405, *The SUPPORT for Patients and Communities Act (P.L. 115-271): Food and Drug Administration and Controlled Substance Provisions*.

[36] U.S. Drug Enforcement Administration (DEA), *Justice Department, DEA propose significant opioid manufacturing reduction in 2019*, August 16, 2018, https://www.dea.gov/press-releases/2018/08/16/justice-department-dea-propose- significant-opioid-manufacturing-reduction.

[37] U.S. Drug Enforcement Administration (DEA), "Established Aggregate Production Quotas for Schedule I and II Controlled Substances and Assessment of Annual Needs for the List I

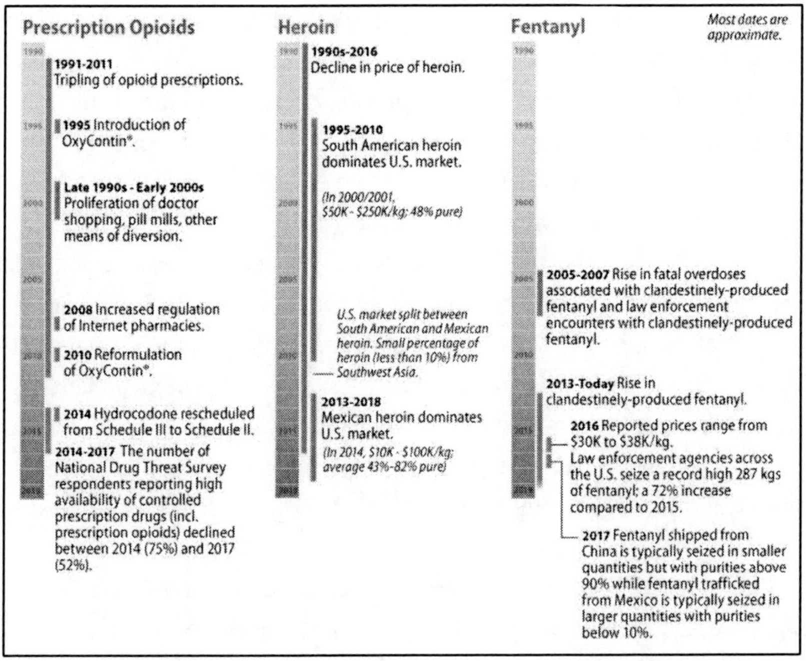

Source: U.S. Department of Justice, Drug Enforcement Administration; National Institute on Drug Abuse; and U.S. Department of Justice, National Drug Intelligence Center.

Notes: Under the Controlled Substances Act, there are five schedules under which substances may be classified—Schedule I being the most restrictive. Substances placed onto one of the five schedules are evaluated on potential for abuse, current scientific knowledge of the substance, risk to public health, and several other criteria. For example, heroin is categorized as a Schedule I drug and has no recognized medical use, while oxycodone and hydrocodone have recognized medical use and are categorized as Schedule II.

Figure 2. Timeline of the Opioid Supply. 1990s-Today.

Heroin Supply

The trajectory of the heroin supply over the last several decades is much different than that of prescription opioids, but their stories are

---

Chemicals Ephedrine, Pseudoephedrine, and Phenylpropanolamine for 2019," 83 *Federal Register* 67348-67354, December 28, 2018.

connected.[38] In the late 1990s and early 2000s, white powder heroin produced in South America dominated the market east of the Mississippi River, and black tar and brown powder heroin produced in Mexico dominated the market west of the Mississippi.[39] Most of the heroin found in the United States at that time came from South America, while smaller percentages came from Mexico and Southwest Asia.

In the 1990s, the purity and price of retail-level heroin varied considerably by region. The average retail-level purity of South American heroin was around 46%, which was considerably higher than that of Mexican, Southeast Asian, or Southwest Asian heroin. Mexican heroin was around 27% pure, while Southeast Asian and Southwest Asian heroin were around 24% and 30% pure, respectively.[40] Retail prices for heroin fell dramatically throughout the 1990s—it was 55% to 65% less expensive in 1999 than in 1989.[41]

Through 2017, retail-level heroin prices continued to decline (although they increased slightly from 2015 to 2016), while purity, in particular that of Mexican heroin, has increased (although purity also dipped slightly from 2015 to 2016).[42] The availability of Mexican heroin has increased. In 2016, nearly 90% of the heroin seized and tested in the United States was determined to have come from Mexico, while a much smaller portion was from South America.[43] Mexican-sourced heroin dominates the U.S. heroin market, in part, because of its proximity and its established transportation and distribution infrastructure. In addition, increases in Mexican production have ensured a reliable supply of low-cost heroin, even as demand for the drug has increased. Mexican transnational criminal

---

[38] U.S. Department of Health and Human Services (HHS), National Institutes of Health (NIH), National Institute on Drug Abuse (NIDA), *Prescription Drugs and Heroin*, December 2015, pp. 4-5.

[39] Heroin has several different forms, including black tar, brown powder, and white powder. For more information, see DEA, *Drugs of Abuse: A DEA Resource Guide, 2017 Edition*, p. 42.

[40] U.S. Department of Justice (DOJ), National Drug Intelligence Center (NDIC), *National Drug Threat Assessment 2005*, February 2005.

[41] Executive Office of the President, Office of National Drug Control Policy, *The Price and Purity of Illicit Drugs: 1981 Through the Second Quarter of 2003*, November 2004, p. 11.

[42] U.S. Drug Enforcement Administration (DEA), *2017 National Drug Threat Assessment*, October 2017; and *2018 National Drug Threat Assessment.*

[43] *2018 National Drug Threat Assessment.*

organizations have particularly increased their production of white powder heroin as they have expanded their retail presence[44] into the eastern part of the United States (where the primary form of heroin consumed has been white powder) and they have diversified the heroin sold in western states. Of further concern is the increasing amount of heroin seizures containing fentanyl and/or fentanyl-related substances.[45]

Fentanyl Supply

Exacerbating the current opioid problem is the rise of illicit nonpharmaceutical fentanyl[46] available on the black market. Diverted pharmaceutical fentanyl represents only a small portion of the fentanyl market. Illicit nonpharmaceutical fentanyl largely comes from China, and it is often mixed with or sold as heroin. It is 50 to 100 times more potent than heroin, and over the last several years, reported prices ranged between $30,000 and $38,000 per kilogram. The increased potency of illicit nonpharmaceutical fentanyl compounds, such as "gray death,"[47] is even more dangerous. Law enforcement expects that illicit fentanyl distributors will continue to create new fentanyl products to circumvent new U.S., Chinese, and Mexican laws and regulations.[48]

Where are Illicit Opioids Produced?

Illicit opioids include those from plant-based and synthetic sources. While some opium poppy crops are legally cultivated to meet global

---

[44] Mexican transnational criminal organizations (TCOs) work with local groups and street gangs for retail-level distribution.

[45] Ibid.

[46] Fentanyl and fentanyl compounds such as acetyl fentanyl and carfentanil are synthetic opioids with varying levels of potency. Fentanyl is a Schedule II narcotic and approved by the FDA. While some pharmaceutical fentanyl is diverted from legitimate use, illicit nonpharmaceutical fentanyl is the largest fentanyl threat in the United States. For more information, see U.S. Drug Enforcement Administration (DEA), *Drugs of Abuse: A DEA Resource Guide, 2017 Edition*, p. 40, and *2018 National Drug Threat Assessment*, pp. 21-37.

[47] Gray death is an illicit synthetic opioid mix that is reportedly 10,000 times more powerful than morphine. The formulations of seized samples have varied.

[48] *2018 National Drug Threat Assessment*, p. vi.

demand for scientific and medicinal purposes, the United Nations (U.N.) estimates that approximately 345,800 hectares of opium poppy crops were illicitly cultivated around the world in 2018—a 16.6% decrease from the estimated 414,500 hectares in 2017.[49] The vast majority of illicit opium poppy is grown in Afghanistan, which cultivated approximately 263,000 hectares in 2018. Most heroin consumed in the United States is derived from illicit opium poppy crops cultivated in Mexico.[50] According to U.S. government estimates, approximately 44,100 hectares of illicit opium poppy was cultivated in Mexico in 2017 (up from 28,000 hectares cultivated in 2015).[51] Illicit cultivation of opium poppy has also been reported in Burma (37,300 hectares in 2018), Laos (5,700 hectares in 2015), and Colombia (282 hectares in 2017). Several dozen other countries have reported comparatively smaller seizures of opium poppy plants and eradication of opium poppy crops.

Synthetic opioids may enter the illicit drug market through diversion from legitimate pharmaceutical manufacturing operations or through the clandestine production of counterfeit medicines and/or of psychoactive substances intended for recreational consumption. Illicit synthetic opioids consumed in the United States are mostly foreign-sourced. According to the State Department, "China's large chemical and pharmaceutical industries provide an ideal environment for the illicit production and export of [synthetic drugs]."[52] The State Department also reports that India's pharmaceutical and chemical industries are particularly susceptible to criminal exploitation; India legally produces opium for pharmaceutical uses and manufactures synthetic opiate pharmaceuticals, in addition to numerous precursor chemicals that could be diverted and used as ingredients in the production of illicit opioids. Clandestine laboratories

---

[49] Unless otherwise noted, opium poppy cultivation statistics in this paragraph are sourced from United Nations Office on Drugs and Crime (UNODC), *World Drug Report 2018*, June 2019.

[50] See CRS In Focus IF10400, *Transnational Crime Issues: Heroin Production, Fentanyl Trafficking, and U.S.-Mexico Security Cooperation*; and 2018 National Drug Threat Assessment, p. 18.

[51] *2018 National Drug Threat Assessment*, p. 18, and U.S. Drug Enforcement Administration, *2016 National Drug Threat Assessment Summary*, p. 54.

[52] U.S. Department of State, *International Narcotics Control Strategy Report* (INCSR), Volume 1, March 2018.

illicitly producing fentanyl have been discovered in Mexico, Canada, the Dominican Republic, the United States, and other countries.[53]

How do Illicit Opioids Enter the Country?

Prescription Opioids

The active and inactive ingredients in prescription opioids may come from various countries around the world.[54] Prescription drugs may be manufactured domestically or abroad. Current law and regulations allow for the importation of certain prescription drugs that are manufactured outside the country.[55] Prescription drugs in the United States, regardless of where they were manufactured, flow through a regulated supply chain[56]—involving manufacturers, processers, packagers, importers, and distributors—until they are ultimately dispensed to end users.

The majority of misused prescription opioids available in the United States have been prescribed for a legitimate use and then diverted. Counterfeit prescription opioids are also available; in these cases, substances have often been pressed into pills in the United States, or abroad and then transported into the country, and sold. The DEA has indicated that one of the reasons traffickers may be disguising other opioids as CPDs could be that they are attempting to "gain access to new users."[57]

---

[53] Ibid. See also "Mexican Officials Bust Fentanyl Lab in Mexico City," *Reuters*, December 13, 2018.

[54] Some reports have indicated that many active ingredients may come from countries such as China and India. See, for example, David Lazarus, "Where Do Prescription Drugs Come From? Good Luck Answering That Question," *Los Angeles Times*, May 15, 2018.

[55] For more information on prescription drug regulation and issues involving prescription drug importation, see CRS In Focus IF11056, *Prescription Drug Importation*.

[56] For more information on the pharmaceutical supply chain, see CRS Report R43106, *Pharmaceutical Supply Chain Security*.

[57] *2018 National Drug Threat Assessment*, p. vi, and 97-99.

Heroin[58]

Mexican transnational criminal organizations (TCOs) are the major suppliers and key producers of most illegal drugs smuggled into the United States,[59] and they have been increasing their share of the U.S. heroin market. The *2018 National Drug Threat Assessment* notes that most illicit heroin flows into the United States over the Southwest border. It is primarily moved through legal ports of entry (POEs) in passenger vehicles or tractor trailers where it can be co-mingled with legal goods; a smaller amount of heroin is seized from individuals carrying the drugs on their person or in backpacks.[60] Data from U.S. Customs and Border Protection (CBP) indicate that in FY2018, 5,205 pounds of heroin were seized at POEs, and 568 pounds were seized between POEs.[61]

Illicitly Produced Fentanyl[62]

The DEA notes that "[f]entanyl continues to be smuggled into the United States primarily in powder or counterfeit pill form, indicating illicitly produced fentanyl as opposed to pharmaceutical fentanyl from the countries of origin."[63] Fentanyl is smuggled into the United States directly from China through the mail,[64] from China through Canada, or across the Southwest border from Mexico.[65] Smaller quantities of fentanyl with

---

[58] For more information on heroin trafficking, see CRS Report R44599, *Heroin Trafficking in the United States*.

[59] *2018 National Drug Threat Assessment*, p. vi.

[60] Ibid.

[61] U.S. Customs and Border Protection, *CBP Enforcement Statistics FY2018*, https://www.cbp.gov/newsroom/stats/cbp- enforcement-statistics.

[62] In this section, references to "fentanyl" mean illicitly produced fentanyl rather than legal pharmaceutical fentanyl, unless otherwise noted.

[63] *2018 National Drug Threat Assessment*, p. 21.

[64] Of note, in trying to counter fentanyl trafficking through the U.S. mail, Section 8003 of the SUPPORT Act required the United States Postal Service (USPS) to ensure transmission of advance electronic data of at least 70% of all inbound international mail and advance electronic data of 100% of inbound international mail from the People's Republic of China by December 31, 2018. By December 31, 2020, USPS is required to provide advance electronic data for 100% of inbound international mail shipments. For broader discussion, see CRS Report R45423, *Public Health and Other Related Provisions in P.L 115-271, the SUPPORT for Patients and Communities Act*.

[65] *2018 National Drug Threat Assessment*, pp. 33-34.

relatively high purity (some over 90%) are smuggled from China, and larger quantities of fentanyl with relatively low purity (often less than 10%) are transported from Mexico.[66] The DEA notes that Mexican traffickers often get fentanyl precursor chemicals from China. In addition, these traffickers may receive fentanyl from China, adulterate it, and smuggle it into the United States.

Data from CBP indicate that in FY2018, 1,785 pounds of fentanyl were seized at POEs, and 388 pounds were seized between POEs.[67] The DEA reports that the San Diego border sector has been the primary entry point for fentanyl coming into the United States across the Southwest border (85% of the fentanyl seized coming across the Southwest border in 2017 flowed through the San Diego sector, and 14% came through the Tucson sector). Most commonly, the fentanyl seized coming through Southwest border POEs was smuggled in personally operated vehicles.[68]

Opioids and Domestic Supply Control Policy

How does the Federal Government Counter Illicit Opioid Trafficking in the United States?[69]

There are a number of federal departments and agencies involved in countering illicit opioid trafficking in the United States.

Office of National Drug Control Policy (ONDCP)

ONDCP is responsible for creating, implementing, and evaluating U.S. drug control policies to reduce the use, manufacturing, and trafficking of illicit drugs as well as drug-related health consequences, crime, and

---

[66] Ibid., p. 33.

[67] U.S. Customs and Border Protection, *CBP Enforcement Statistics FY2018*, https://www.cbp.gov/newsroom/stats/cbp- enforcement-statistics.

[68] *2018 National Drug Threat Assessment.*

[69] This report does not discuss the roles of all federal agencies involved in countering illicit opioid trafficking.

violence.[70] The ONDCP director is required to develop a National Drug Control Strategy (Strategy) to direct the nation's anti-drug efforts and a National Drug Control Budget (Budget) designed to implement the Strategy. The director also is required to coordinate implementation of the policies, goals, objectives, and priorities established by the Administration by agencies contributing to the Federal Drug Control Program.[71] In addition, ONDCP manages several grant programs, including the High Intensity Drug Trafficking Areas (HIDTA) program.[72] While ONDCP is not focused solely on countering opioid-related threats, it is a major priority of the office.[73]

HIDTA

The HIDTA program provides assistance to law enforcement agencies—at the federal, state, local, and tribal levels—that are operating in regions of the United States that have been deemed critical drug trafficking areas. There are 29 designated HIDTAs throughout the United States and its territories. The program aims to reduce drug production and trafficking through four means:

- promoting coordination and information sharing between federal, state, local, and tribal law enforcement;
- bolstering intelligence sharing between federal, state, local, and tribal law enforcement;
- providing reliable intelligence to law enforcement agencies such that they may be better equipped to design effective enforcement operations and strategies; and

---

[70] For more information on ONDCP, see CRS Report R45423, *Public Health and Other Related Provisions in P.L 115-271, the SUPPORT for Patients and Communities Act.*

[71] 21 U.S.C. §1703.

[72] For more information about the HIDTA program, see CRS Report R45188, *High Intensity Drug Trafficking Areas (HIDTA) Program.* See also Executive Office of the President, Office of National Drug Control Policy, *High Intensity Drug Trafficking Areas (HIDTA) Program.*

[73] See, for example, https://www.whitehouse.gov/ondcp/key-issues/prescription-opioid-misuse/.

- promoting coordinated law enforcement strategies that rely upon available resources to reduce illegal drug supplies, not only in a given area but throughout the country.[74]

HIDTA funds can be used to support the most pressing drug trafficking threats in the region. As such, when heroin trafficking is found to be a top priority in a HIDTA region, funds may be used to support initiatives targeting it.

In addition, in 2015 ONDCP launched the Heroin Response Strategy (HRS), "a multi-HIDTA, cross-disciplinary approach that develops partnerships among public safety and public health agencies at the Federal, state, and local levels to reduce drug overdose fatalities and disrupt trafficking in illicit opioids."[75] Within the HRS, a Public Health and Public Safety Network coordinates teams of public health analysts and drug intelligence officers in each state. The HRS not only provides information to these participating entities on drug trafficking and use, but it has "developed and disseminated prevention activities, including a parent helpline and online materials."[76]

Other ONDCP Supply Control Initiatives

ONDCP has been involved in various other counter-trafficking operations since its creation in 1988.[77] Recently, it collaborated with the U.S. Department of Homeland Security's Science and Technology Directorate (as well as CBP and the U.S. Postal Inspection Service) to

---

[74] 21 U.S.C. §1706(a)(2).

[75] Executive Office of the President, Office of National Drug Control Policy, Heroin Response Strategy, Annual Program Report for 2016, May 2, 2017, p. 1.

[76] Ibid.

[77] One example is the Counterdrug Technology Assessment Center (CTAC). One of CTAC's programs was the Technology Transfer Program, which supported state and local law enforcement agencies' counterdrug missions through technology and training. The CTAC program was discontinued in FY2011. For more information on CTAC and its creation and cancellation, see Office of National Drug Control Policy (ONDCP), *National Drug Control Strategy: Budget Summary*, February 1994, p. 123; and ONDCP, *National Drug Control Strategy: FY2011 Budget Summary*, 2010, p. 149.

launch the Opioid Detection Challenge—a $1.55 million global prize competition to seek new solutions to detect opioids in international mail.[78]

Department of Justice (DOJ)

DOJ controls the opioid supply through law enforcement; regulation of manufacturers, distributors, and dispensers; and grants to state and local agencies. U.S. efforts to target opioid trafficking have centered on law enforcement initiatives.

There are a number of DOJ law enforcement agencies involved in countering opioid trafficking. Within these agencies, there are a range of activities aimed at (or that may be tailored to) curbing opioid trafficking.

Organized Crime Drug Enforcement Task Force (OCDETF) Program

The OCDETF program targets—with the intent to disrupt and dismantle—major drug trafficking and money laundering organizations. Federal agencies that participate in the OCDETF program include the DEA; Federal Bureau of Investigation (FBI); Bureau of Alcohol, Tobacco, Firearms, and Explosives (ATF); U.S. Marshals; Internal Revenue Service (IRS); U.S. Immigration and Customs Enforcement (ICE); U.S. Coast Guard; Offices of the U.S. Attorneys; and the Department of Justice's (DOJ's) Criminal Division. These federal agencies also collaborate with state and local law enforcement on task forces.[79] There are 14 OCDETF strike forces around the country and an OCDETF Fusion Center that gathers and analyzes intelligence and information to support OCDETF operations. The OCDETFs target those organizations that have been identified on the Consolidated Priority Organization Targets (CPOT) List, the "most wanted" list for leaders of drug trafficking and money laundering organizations. During FY2018, 52% of active OCDETF investigations involved heroin. According to DOJ, "OCDETF has adjusted

---

[78] The competition deadline was April 24, 2019. For more information, see https://www.opioiddetectionchallenge.com/.

[79] U.S. Department of Justice, Organized Crime Drug Enforcement Task Forces, *FY 2020 Interagency Crime and Drug Enforcement President's Budget*.

its resources to target these investigations in an attempt to reduce the [heroin] supply."[80]

Drug Enforcement Administration (DEA)

The DEA enforces federal controlled substances laws in all states and territories. The agency has developed a 360 Strategy aimed at "tackling the cycle of violence and addiction generated by the link between drug cartels, violent gangs, and the rising problem of prescription opioid and heroin abuse."[81] The 360 Strategy leverages federal, state, and local law enforcement, diversion control, and community outreach organizations to achieve its goals. Additionally, the DEA routinely uses community-based enforcement strategies as well as multijurisdictional task forces to address opioid trafficking.[82]

The DEA also operates a heroin signature program (HSP) and a heroin domestic monitor program (HDMP) to identify the geographic sources of heroin seized in the United States. The HSP analyzes wholesale-level samples of "heroin seized at U.S. ports of entry (POEs), all non-POE heroin exhibits weighing more than one kilogram, randomly chosen samples, and special requests for analysis."[83] The HDMP samples retail-level heroin seized in selected cities across the country.[84] Chemical analysis of a given heroin sample can identify its "signature," which indicates a particular heroin production process that has been linked to a specific geographic region. In addition, the DEA has started a Fentanyl Signature Profiling Program (FSPP), analyzing samples from fentanyl seizures to help "identify the international and domestic trafficking networks responsible for many of the drugs fueling the opioid crisis."[85]

---

[80] Ibid., p. 21.

[81] U.S. Drug Enforcement Administration (DEA), *DEA 360 Strategy: Working Together to Break the Cycle of Drug Trafficking, Drug Violence, and Drug Abuse*, p. 1.

[82] U.S. Drug Enforcement Administration (DEA), *360 Strategy—Law Enforcement*, https://admin.dea.gov/360- strategy-law-enforcement.

[83] U.S. Drug Enforcement Administration (DEA), *The 2016 Heroin Signature Program Report*, October 2018, p. 2.

[84] U.S. Drug Enforcement Administration (DEA), *FY 2019 Performance Budget Congressional Submission.*

[85] Ibid., p. 47.

Federal Bureau of Investigation (FBI)

The FBI investigates opioid trafficking as part of its efforts to counter transnational organized crime and gangs, cybercriminals, fraudsters, and other malicious actors. The FBI participates in investigations that range from targeting drug distribution networks bringing opioids across the Southwest border[86] to prioritizing illicit opioid distributors leveraging the Dark Web[87] to sell their drugs.[88]

Other DOJ Agencies

Other DOJ agencies have key roles in combatting the opioid epidemic. The Offices of the U.S. Attorneys are responsible for the prosecution of federal criminal and civil cases, which include cases against prescribers, pharmaceutical companies, and pharmacies involved in unlawful manufacturing, distribution, and dispensing of opioids as well as illicit opioid traffickers. Other enforcement agencies such as the ATF and U.S. Marshals may also be involved in seizing illicit opioids in the course of carrying out their official duties. The Office of Justice Programs (OJP) administers grant programs to address opioid supply and demand (some of which are discussed below in "Which DOJ grant programs may be used to address the opioid epidemic?").

U.S. Department of Homeland Security (DHS)

U.S. Customs and Border Protection (CBP)

CBP works to counter the trafficking of illicit opioids (among other drugs) along the U.S. borders as well as via mail curriers. To help detect and interdict these substances, CBP employs tools such as nonintrusive inspection equipment (including x-ray and imaging systems), canines, and laboratory testing of suspicious substances. The agency also uses

---

[86] See, for example, Department of Justice, "20 Individuals Charged with Trafficking Heroin and Fentanyl," press release, December 13, 2016.

[87] For more information on the Dark Web, see CRS Report R44101, *Dark Web*.

[88] See, for example, Department of Justice, "Attorney General Jeff Sessions Announces Results of J-Code's First Law Enforcement Operation Targeting Opioid Trafficking on the Darknet," press release, April 3, 2018.

information and screening systems to help detect illicit drugs, targeting precursor chemicals, equipment, and the drugs themselves.[89]

CBP, through the Office of Field Operations (OFO) and the U.S. Border Patrol, seizes illicit drugs coming into the United States at and between POEs.[90] CBP data indicate that 90% of the heroin seized by CBP in FY2018 was seized by OFO at POEs, and 10% was seized by the Border Patrol between POEs. In addition, these data indicate that 82% of the fentanyl seized in FY2018 was seized by OFO at POEs, and 18% was seized by the Border Patrol between POEs.[91]

U.S. Coast Guard (USCG)

Drug interdiction is part of the Coast Guard's law enforcement mission. The agency is responsible for interdicting noncommercial maritime flows of illegal drugs. Cocaine is the primary illicit drug encountered by the Coast Guard, as it is the most common drug moved via noncommercial vessels.[92] While the Coast Guard encounters other illicit drugs, including opioids, the agency notes that those drugs are more commonly moved on land or in commercial maritime vessels that are regulated by other enforcement agencies.[93] The Coast Guard also participates in multi-agency counterdrug task forces, including OCDETF.

U.S. Postal Inspection Service (USPIS)

USPIS is the law enforcement arm of the U.S. Postal Service. It shares responsibility for international mail security with other federal agencies, and as a result of the opioid epidemic, it has dedicated more resources to investigating prohibited substances in the mail.[94] From FY2016 through FY2018, USPIS had a "1,000% increase in international parcel seizures

---

[89] Testimony of Casey Owen Durst, U.S. Customs and Border Protection, before U.S. Congress, House Committee on Homeland Security, Subcommittee on Oversight and Management Efficiency, *Combating Opioid Smuggling*, 115th Cong., 2nd sess., June 19, 2018.

[90] Ports of entry include land, air, and sea POEs.

[91] Data are available at https://www.cbp.gov/newsroom/stats/cbp-enforcement-statistics.

[92] United States Coast Guard, *United States Coast Guard Annual Performance Report: Fiscal Year 2017*, p. 14.

[93] Ibid.

[94] U.S. Postal Inspection Service, *Annual Report FY2018*, p. 5.

and a 750% increase in domestic parcel seizures related to opioids."[95] In FY2018, USPIS and its law enforcement partners seized over 96,000 pounds of drugs in the mail, including marijuana, methamphetamine, synthetic opioids, and others, but their publicly available data does not describe what portion of these drugs were opioids.[96]

What is the DEA's Role in Preventing the Diversion of Prescription Opioids?

The DEA has a key regulatory function in drug control. While it conducts traditional law enforcement activities such as investigating drug trafficking (including trafficking of heroin and other illicit opioids), it also regulates the flow of controlled substances in the United States. The Controlled Substances Act (CSA)[97] requires the DEA to establish and maintain a closed system of distribution for controlled substances; this involves the regulation of anyone who handles controlled substances, including exporters, importers, manufacturers, distributors, health care professionals, pharmacists, and researchers.

Unless specifically exempted by the CSA, these individuals must register with the DEA. Registrants must keep records of all transactions involving controlled substances, maintain detailed inventories of the substances in their possession, and periodically file reports with the DEA, as well as ensure that controlled substances are securely stored and safeguarded.[98] The DEA regulates over 1.5 million registrants.[99]

---

[95] Ibid., p. 20.

[96] Ibid. Annual reports from 2016 and 2017 were unavailable from USPIS at the time this report was published. CRS relies on the statement made by USPIS to describe the increase, but the volume of drugs seized in previous years remains unclear.

[97] The Controlled Substances Act (CSA), enacted as Title II of the Comprehensive Drug Abuse Prevention and Control Act of 1970 (P.L. 91-513), placed the control of select plants, drugs, and chemical substances under federal jurisdiction.

[98] For more details on the CSA regulatory requirements, see CRS Report RL34635, *The Controlled Substances Act: Regulatory Requirements* (available to congressional clients upon request).

[99] U.S. Congress, House Committee on Energy and Commerce, *Improving Predictability and Transparency in DEA and FDA Regulation*, Statement of Joseph T. Rannazzisi, Deputy

The DEA uses its criminal, civil, and administrative authorities to maintain a closed system of distribution and prevent diversion of drugs, such as prescription opioids, from legitimate purposes. Actions include inspections, order form requirements, education, and establishing quotas for Schedule I and II controlled substances.[100] More severe administrative actions include immediate suspension orders and orders to show cause for registrations.[101] As noted previously, in 2018 the DEA significantly lowered the aggregate production quota for opioids in 2019.[102]

Which DOJ Grant Programs may be Used to Address the Opioid Epidemic?

Discussed below are grant programs that have a direct or possible avenue to address the opioid epidemic. This discussion provides examples of such programs, and should not be considered exhaustive. Many DOJ grant programs have broad purpose areas for which funds can be used. While some focus on broad crime reduction strategies that might include efforts to combat drug- related crime, others—including the selected

---

Assistant Administrator, Office of Diversion Control, Drug Enforcement Administration, 113th Cong., 2nd sess., April 7, 2014, p. 1.

[100] Under the Controlled Substances Act (CSA), there are five schedules under which substances may be classified— Schedule I being the most restrictive. Substances placed onto one of the five schedules are evaluated on potential for abuse, current scientific knowledge of the substance, risk to public health, and several other criteria. Of the more well- known opioids, heroin is categorized as a Schedule I drug, while oxycodone and hydrocodone have recognized medical use and are categorized as Schedule II. Per the CSA and regulation, the DEA establishes quotas to limit the quantity of Schedule I and II controlled substances that may be produced in a given calendar year. For more information on CSA regulations, see CRS Report RL34635, *The Controlled Substances Act: Regulatory Requirements* (available to congressional clients upon request).

[101] See 21 C.F.R. §§1301.36 and 1301.37. The DEA administrator may issue an immediate suspension order that suspends a registrant's DEA registration, and may do so simultaneously with an order to show cause proceeding if the continued registration (pending the administrative proceeding) would pose an imminent danger to public health or safety.

[102] U.S. Drug Enforcement Administration (DEA), "Established Aggregate Production Quotas for Schedule I and II Controlled Substances and Assessment of Annual Needs for the List I Chemicals Ephedrine, Pseudoephedrine, and Phenylpropanolamine for 2019," 83 *Federal Register* 67348-67354, December 28, 2018.

programs—have purpose areas that are more specifically focused on drug threats. Of note, these programs do not solely address illicit drug supply control; some also address demand as well as other criminal justice issues. They are included because they are administered by DOJ agencies.

Comprehensive Opioid Abuse Grant Program (COAP)

COAP is a recently created DOJ grant program[103] (administered by BJA) for states, units of local government, and Indian tribes (34 U.S.C. 10701 et seq.). This grant program supports projects primarily relating to opioid abuse, including (1) diversion and alternatives to incarceration projects; (2) collaboration between criminal justice, social service, and substance abuse agencies; (3) overdose outreach projects, including law enforcement training related to overdoses; (4) strategies to support those with a history of opioid misuse,[104] including justice-involved individuals; (5) prescription drug monitoring programs; (6) development of interventions based on a public health and public safety understanding of opioid abuse; and (7) planning and implementation of comprehensive strategies in response to the growing opioid epidemic.[105]

The Harold Rogers Prescription Drug Monitoring Program (PDMP) was incorporated into COAP. The Harold Rogers PDMP is a competitive grant program that was created to help law enforcement, regulatory entities, and public health officials collect and analyze data on prescriptions for controlled substances. Law enforcement uses of PDMP

---

[103] Section 201 of the Comprehensive Addiction and Recovery Act of 2016 (CARA; P.L. 114-198) amended Title I of the Omnibus Crime Control and Safe Streets Act of 1968 to authorize the program, and the Reauthorizing and Extending Grants for Recovery From Opioid Use Programs (REGROUP) Act of 2018 (Sections 8091-8092 of the SUPPORT Act) reauthorized funding for the COAP through FY2023.

[104] Grantees may develop and implement strategies "to identify and provide treatment and recovery support services to 'high frequency' utilizers of multiple systems (e.g., health care, child welfare, criminal justice, etc.) who have a history of opioid misuse." See BJA, *FY17 Comprehensive Opioid Abuse Site-based Program Awards: Category 4: Statewide Planning, Coordination, and Implementation Projects*, p. 1, https://www.bja.gov/ funding/ Category-4-awards.pdf.

[105] For more information on the Comprehensive Opioid Abuse Site-based Program, see U.S. Department of Justice, Office of Justice Programs, Bureau of Justice Assistance, *Comprehensive Opioid Abuse Program*, https://www.bja.gov/ ProgramDetails.aspx?Program_ID=72.

data include (but are not limited to) investigations of physicians who prescribe controlled substances for drug dealers or abusers, pharmacists who falsify records in order to sell controlled substances, and people who forge prescriptions.[106]

COPS Anti-Heroin Task Force Program

The Community Oriented Policing Services (COPS) Office's Anti-Heroin Task Force (AHTF) Program provides funding assistance on a competitive basis to state law enforcement agencies to investigate illicit activities related to the trafficking or distribution of heroin or diverted prescription opioids. Funds are distributed to states with high rates of primary treatment admissions for heroin and other opioids. Further, the program focuses its funding on state law enforcement agencies with multi-jurisdictional reach and interdisciplinary team structures—such as task forces.[107]

Drug Courts[108]

The Drug Court Discretionary Grant Program

The Drug Court Discretionary Grant program[109] (Drug Courts Program) is meant to enhance drug court services, coordination, and substance abuse treatment and recovery support services. It is a BJA-administered, competitive grant program that provides resources to state, local, and tribal courts and governments to enhance drug court programs for nonviolent substance-abusing offenders. Drug courts are designed to help reduce recidivism and substance abuse among participants and increase an offender's likelihood of successful rehabilitation through early,

---

[106] The conditions under which law enforcement may access state PDMP data is determined by state law. For more information about PDMPs, see CRS Report R42593, *Prescription Drug Monitoring Programs*.

[107] U.S. Department of Justice (DOJ), Community Oriented Policing Services (COPS), *Fact Sheet: 2018 COPS Anti- Heroin Task Force Program*.

[108] For more information on drug courts, see CRS Report R44467, *Federal Support for Drug Courts: In Brief*.

[109] 34 U.S.C. §§10611-10619.

continuous, and intense judicially supervised treatment; mandatory periodic drug testing; community supervision; appropriate sanctions; and other rehabilitation services.

The Drug Courts Program is not focused on opioid abusers, but drug-involved offenders, including opioids abusers, may be processed through drug courts.

Veterans Treatment Courts

BJA administers the Veterans Treatment Court Program through the Drug Courts Program using funds specifically appropriated for this purpose. The purpose of the Veterans Treatment Court Program is "to serve veterans struggling with addiction, serious mental illness, and/or co-occurring disorders."[110] Grants are awarded to state, local, and tribal governments to fund the establishment and development of veterans treatment courts. While veterans treatment court grants have been part of the OJP's Drug Courts Program for several years, the Comprehensive Addiction and Recovery Act of 2016 (CARA; P.L. 114-198) authorized DOJ to award grants to state, local, and tribal governments to establish or expand programs for qualified veterans,[111] including veterans treatment courts; peer-to-peer services; and treatment, rehabilitation, legal, or transitional services for incarcerated veterans.[112]

Juvenile and Family Drug Treatment Courts

The Office of Juvenile Justice and Delinquency Prevention (OJJDP) supports juvenile and family drug court programs through its Drug Treatment Courts Program. This program supports the implementation or enhancement of state, local, and tribal drug court programs that focus on juveniles and parents with substance abuse issues. One of its specific goals

---

[110] U.S. Department of Justice (DOJ), Office of Justice Programs (OJP), *FY2017 Performance Budget*, p. 51, https://www.justice.gov/jmd/file/822366/download.

[111] CARA defines a qualified veteran as a preliminarily qualified offender who served on active duty in any branch of the Armed Forces, including the National Guard or Reserves, and was discharged or released from such service under conditions other than dishonorable, unless the reason for the dishonorable discharge was attributable to a substance abuse disorder.

[112] For more information on veterans treatment courts, see CRS Report R44467, *Federal Support for Drug Courts: In Brief*.

is to help those with substance abuse problems related to opioid abuse or co-occurring mental health disorders who are involved with the court system.[113]

The Edward Byrne Memorial Justice Assistance Grant (JAG) Program

Administered by BJA, the JAG program provides funding to state, local, and tribal governments for state and local initiatives, technical assistance, training, personnel, equipment, supplies, contractual support, and criminal justice information systems in eight program purpose areas: (1) law enforcement programs; (2) prosecution and court programs; (3) prevention and education programs; (4) corrections and community corrections programs; (5) drug treatment and enforcement programs; (6) planning, evaluation, and technology improvement programs; (7) crime victim and witness programs (other than compensation); and (8) mental health and related law enforcement and corrections programs, including behavioral programs and crisis intervention teams. Given the breadth of the program, funds could be used for opioid abuse programs, but state and local governments that receive JAG funds are not required to use their funding for this purpose.[114]

Justice and Mental Health Collaboration Program (JMHCP)

Also administered by BJA, the JMHCP supports collaborative criminal justice and mental health systems efforts to assist individuals with mental illnesses or co-occurring mental health and substance abuse disorders who come into contact with the justice system. It encourages early intervention for these individuals; supports training for justice and treatment professionals; and facilitates collaborative support services among justice professionals, treatment and related service providers, and governmental partners. Three types of grants are supported under this program: (1)

---

[113] See current and past OJJDP grant solicitations for the Drug Treatment Courts Program for additional details.

[114] For more information on the Byrne-JAG Program, see U.S. Department of Justice (DOJ), Office of Justice Programs (OJP), Bureau of Justice Assistance (BJA), *Edward Byrne Memorial Justice Assistance Grant (JAG) Program*, https://www.bja.gov/jag/.

Collaborative County Approaches to Reducing the Prevalence of Individuals with Mental Disorders in Jail, (2) Planning and Implementation, and (3) Expansion.[115]

Juvenile Justice Program Grants

Juvenile Justice and Delinquency Prevention Act (JJDPA) Formula Grant Program

The JJDPA authorizes OJJDP to make formula grants[116] to states that can be used to fund the planning, establishment, operation, coordination, and evaluation of projects for the development of more-effective juvenile delinquency programs and improved juvenile justice systems. Funds provided to the state may be used for a wide array of juvenile justice related programs, such as substance abuse prevention and treatment programs. None of the program purpose areas deal specifically with combating opioid abuse, but they are broad enough that the grants made under this program could be used for this purpose.

JJDPA Title V Incentive Grants Program

The JJDPA authorizes OJJDP to make discretionary grants[117] to the states that are then transmitted to units of local government in order to carry out delinquency prevention programs for juveniles who have come into contact, or are likely to come into contact, with the juvenile justice system. Purpose areas include (but are not limited to) alcohol and substance abuse prevention services, educational programs, and child and adolescent health (as well as mental health) services. None of the program purpose areas deal specifically with combating opioid abuse, but they are broad enough that they could be used for this purpose.

---

[115] For more information on this program, see U.S. Department of Justice (DOJ), Office of Justice Programs (OJP), Bureau of Justice Assistance (BJA), *Justice and Mental Health Collaboration Program (JMHCP)*, https://www.bja.gov/ProgramDetails.aspx?Program_ID=66.

[116] 34 U.S.C. §11131 et seq.

[117] 34 U.S.C. §11311 et seq.

Opioid Affected Youth Initiative

The Opioid Affected Youth Initiative is a competitive grant program administered by OJJDP that funds state, local, and tribal government efforts to "develop a data-driven coordinated response to identify and address challenges resulting from opioid abuse that are impacting youth and community safety."[118] The program supports recipients in implementing strategies and programs to identify areas of concern, collect and interpret data to help develop youth strategies and programming, and implement services to assist children, youth, and families affected by opioid abuse.

Residential Substance Abuse Treatment (RSAT) for State Prisoners Program

The RSAT Program is a formula grant program administered by BJA that supports state, local, and tribal governments in developing and implementing substance abuse treatment programs in correctional and detention facilities. Funds may also be used to support reintegration services for offenders as they reenter the community after a period of incarceration. Beginning in FY2018, BJA requires potential grantees to explain "how funded programs will address the addition of opioid abuse reduction treatment and services."[119]

Tribal Resources Grant Program

The COPS Office administers the Tribal Resources Grant Program. It generally supports tribal law enforcement needs, and specifically aims to enhance tribal law enforcement's capacity to engage in anti-opioid activities, among other objectives.[120]

---

[118] U.S. Department of Justice, Office of Juvenile Justice and Delinquency Prevention (OJJDP), *OJJDP FY2019 Opioid Affected Youth Initiative.*

[119] See U.S. Department of Justice (DOJ), Office of Justice Programs (OJP), Bureau of Justice Assistance (BJA), *Residential Substance Abuse Treatment (RSAT) for State Prisoners Program FY2019 Formula Grant Announcement*, p. 9, https://www.bja.gov/funding/RSAT19.pdf.

[120] For more information, see U.S. Department of Justice (DOJ), *U.S. Department of Justice Coordinated Tribal Assistance Solicitation: Fiscal Year 2019 competitive grant announcement*, https://www.justice.gov/tribal/page/file/1114606/download.

Where can DOJ Opioid-Related Grant Funding Information be Found?

For state-specific information on grants and funding from OJP, see the OJP Award Data web page[121] and search by location or by grant solicitation. In FY2018, the Department of Justice released a document entitled, *Fact Sheet: Justice Department is Awarding Almost $320 Million to Combat Opioid Crisis*, which provides a list of FY2018 grantees.[122]

OPIOIDS AND FOREIGN SUPPLY CONTROL POLICY

How does the United States Respond to International Illicit Opioid Trafficking?

The United States has taken a multipronged foreign policy approach to addressing foreign flows of illicit opioids destined for the United States. To date, this approach has included multilateral diplomacy, bilateral efforts, and unilateral action.

On the multilateral front, the U.S. government, primarily working through the U.S. Department of State, engages international organizations and entities involved in addressing drug control issues, including opioids. This includes diplomatic engagement with United Nations (U.N.) entities such as the Commission on Narcotic Drugs (CND), the primary U.N. counternarcotics policy decisionmaking body; the International Narcotics Control Board (INCB), which monitors how member states implement treaty commitments related to drug control; and the U.N. Office of Drugs and Crime (UNODC), mandated to provide technical cooperation and research and analytical projects that support member states' implementation of counternarcotics policies. The United States also addresses opioid trafficking through the Organization of American States'

---

[121] See https://ojp.gov/funding/Explore/OJPAwardData.htm.
[122] See https://www.bja.gov/Programs/FS-Opioids-Substance-Abuse-2018_508.pdf.

(OAS') Inter-American Drug Abuse Control Commission (CICAD). Through such organizations, the United States supports efforts to promote cross-border information sharing.

One objective of U.S. efforts at the U.N. is to accelerate the rate at which new drugs and related precursor chemicals are incorporated into the U.N. international drug control regime. For example, U.S. diplomats advocated for the international control of two of the key chemical precursors used in the production of fentanyl: N-phenethyl-4-piperidone (NPP) and 4-anilino-N- phenethyl-4-piperidone (ANPP). The CND subsequently added NPP and ANPP to the U.N.'s list of drugs and chemicals under international control, effective October 2017.[123]

Until recently, the United States had also engaged the Universal Postal Union (UPU) on the issue of opioid trafficking through international mail. Through the UPU, the United States had, for example, supported the exchange of advance electronic data (AED) for international mail items specifically to improve global efforts to detect and interdict synthetic drugs shipped through the mail.[124] In October 2018, however, the Trump Administration announced that it would begin a one-year withdrawal process from the UPU, potentially affecting how the United States and the UPU engage on opioid matters.[125]

---

[123] International Narcotics Control Board, *INCB: Scheduling of fentanyl precursors comes into force*, press release, October 18, 2017, https://www.incb.org/incb/en/news/press-releases/2017/press_release_20171018.html.

[124] As part of the U.S. government's efforts to collect and exchange advance electronic data (AED) for international mail items, the U.S. Postal Service (USPS) has entered into bilateral agreements with foreign postal operators. Other countries have committed to enter into voluntary data sharing agreements. The USPS also engages foreign counterparts on the exchange of AED through the Kahala Posts Group (KPG), an international alliance of several large-volume postal operators that includes China. See S.Hrg. 115-317, U.S. Senate Permanent Subcommittee on Investigations of the Committee on Homeland Security and Governmental Affairs, "Combatting the Opioid Crisis: Exploiting Vulnerabilities in International Mail," January 25, 2018; and Robert Cintron, Vice President, Network Operations, USPS, prepared testimony for a hearing of the U.S. House of Representatives Subcommittee on Trade of the Committee on Ways and Means, April 25, 2018.

[125] White House (Trump Administration), Statement from the Press Secretary, October 17, 2018, https://www.whitehouse.gov/briefings-statements/statement-press-secretary-38/. An August 23, 2018, Presidential Memorandum had demanded reforms. See White House (Trump Administration), Presidential Memorandum for the Secretary of State, Secretary of the Treasury, Secretary of Homeland Security, Postmaster General, and Chairman of the Postal Regulatory Commission, August 23, 2018, https://www.whitehouse.gov/presidential-

Role of the State Department's Bureau of International Narcotics and Law Enforcement Affairs (INL)

Whether multilaterally or bilaterally, the U.S. Department of State, particularly through the INL Bureau, broadly aims to support and build foreign capacity to disrupt the flow of opioids and other illicit narcotics into the United States.[126] This includes the provision of technical assistance in illicit substances detection, forensics, and cyber investigation techniques as well as sharing with international partners U.S. expertise on reducing drug demand. INL leads the U.S. delegation to the CND and supports projects of the INCB and UNODC with foreign assistance funding appropriated through the International Narcotics Control and Law Enforcement (INCLE) foreign operations account.

INL uses its INCLE funds to train foreign officials to identify and detect illicit substances. This includes providing foreign governments with specialized training to intercept suspicious drugs and chemicals sold online and shipped through the mail and express consignments. INL also funds training and technical assistance programs designed to help foreign governments investigate, prosecute, and dismantle the sale of synthetic drugs online as well as follow the digital money trail of synthetic drug traffickers.[127]

INL also supports demand reduction efforts to promote best practices for the prevention and treatment of drug use.

This includes support for public health messaging on the risks of synthetics; assistance to foreign governments with implementing evidence-based prevention, treatment, and recovery support services; and the development of data collection on the illicit synthetic drug market, including consumption trends, toxicological screening of synthetic drug profiles, and the prevalence of toxic adulterants in illicit drug supplies.[128]

---

actions/presidential- memorandum-secretary-state-secretary-treasury-secretary-homeland-security-postmaster-general-chairman-postal- regulatory-commission/.

[126] U.S. Department of State, Bureau of International Narcotics and Law Enforcement Affairs (INL), *Addressing the Opioid Crisis*, webpage, https://www.state.gov/j/inl/opioid/index.htm.

[127] Kirsten D. Madison, INL Assistant Secretary of State, State Department, prepared testimony for a hearing of the U.S. Senate Caucus on International Drug Control, October 2, 2018. See also Secretary Madison's prepared testimony for a hearing of the U.S. House of Representatives Committee on Foreign Affairs, Subcommittee on Africa, Global Health, Global Human Rights and International Organizations, September 6, 2018.

[128] Ibid.

Bilateral cooperation on opioids has included focused efforts in China, Mexico, and Canada, among other countries. Such engagement has variously taken the form of structured diplomatic dialogues, bilateral law enforcement cooperation, and foreign assistance programming. With respect to China, bilateral cooperation on counternarcotics matters is a top diplomatic priority for the United States.[129]

As with China, U.S. officials pursue bilateral cooperation with Mexico on counternarcotics matters through meetings, including through the cabinet-level U.S.-Mexico Strategic Dialogue on Disrupting Transnational Criminal Organizations, sub-cabinet level U.S.-Mexico Security Cooperation Group, U.S.-Mexico Bilateral Drug Policy Working Group, and National Fentanyl Conference for Forensic Chemists. Trilaterally, the United States, Mexico, and Canada have met several times through the North American Drug Dialogue to address heroin and fentanyl issues. In addition to structured dialogues, U.S. federal law enforcement agencies also engage regularly with their counterparts on ongoing investigations through their representatives based at U.S. embassies and consulates abroad; formal law enforcement cooperation is also facilitated through mutual legal assistance mechanisms.[130]

The United States also funds and conducts programming with China and Mexico to address opioids. In China, INL funding supports drug-related information exchanges, training for Chinese counterparts on specialized topics related to synthetic opioids, and efforts to promote effective drug demand reduction. INL also funds a Resident Legal Advisor, a DOJ prosecutor who is based at the U.S. Embassy in Beijing; a key

---

[129] See CRS In Focus IF10890, *Illicit Fentanyl, China's Role, and U.S. Foreign Policy Options*.

[130] For the past three decades, for example, the DEA has maintained a liaison presence in China. Through DEA's Mexico City country office, it co-leads a Heroin Fentanyl Working Group (HFWG) and implements a U.S.-Mexico bilateral heroin strategy to increase intelligence sharing, coordination of investigations, training, sharing of forensic information, and the control of precursor chemicals. Other U.S. law enforcement agencies represented in China and Mexico include the FBI, as well as the Department of Homeland Security's Immigration and Customs Enforcement Homeland Security Investigations (ICE-HSI) and CBP. See also the prepared testimonies of Paul E. Knierim, Deputy Chief of Operations, Office of Global Enforcement, DEA, and Matthew C. Allen, Assistant Director, Domestic Operations, ICE-HSI, prepared for a hearing of the U.S. Senate Caucus on International Narcotics Control, October 2, 2018.

project has been to conduct outreach to Chinese counterparts involved in amending China's legal and regulatory framework to place the entire fentanyl class of substances under drug control.[131] In Mexico, current efforts to address illicit opioids fit within a broader context of longstanding U.S.-Mexico cooperation to disrupt drug production, dismantle drug distribution networks, prosecute drug traffickers, and deny transnational criminal organizations access to illicit revenue.[132] In such efforts, U.S. support has included programming to address illicit opium poppy cultivation and eradication, drug production and trafficking, border security, and criminal justice judicial institution reform.

In addition, the U.S. government has taken domestic action to address foreign sources and traffickers of opioids through the U.S. criminal justice system and through the application of financial sanctions against specially designated foreign nationals.[133] Recent DOJ indictments have involved Chinese nationals allegedly involved in fentanyl production.[134] Further targeting one of the Chinese nationals under indictment, Jian Zhang, the U.S. Department of the Treasury designated Zhang, four of his associates, and an entity used as a front for the trafficking of fentanyl and fentanyl analogues for sanction, pursuant to the Foreign Narcotics Kingpin Designation Act (Kingpin Act).[135] The Treasury and DOJ have taken

---

[131] Kirsten D. Madison, INL Assistant Secretary of State, State Department, prepared testimony for a hearing of the U.S. Senate Caucus on International Drug Control, October 2, 2018.

[132] See CRS In Focus IF10578, *Mexico: Evolution of the Mérida Initiative, 2007-2019*.

[133] Paul E. Knierim, Deputy Chief of Operations, Office of Global Enforcement, U.S. Drug Enforcement Administration (DEA), prepared testimony for a hearing of the U.S. Senate Caucus on International Narcotics Control, October 2, 2018.

[134] See U.S. Department of Justice (DOJ), "Justice Department Announces First Ever Indictment Against Designated Chinese Manufacturers of Deadly Fentanyl and Other Opiate Substances," press release, October 17, 2017; "Two Chinese Nationals Charged with Operating Global Opioid and Drug Manufacturing Conspiracy Resulting in Deaths," press release, August 22, 2018; and "Chinese National Living in Massachusetts Arrested and Charged with Distributing Opioids that were Shipped from China to the U.S. and Ultimately to Ohio," press release, July 24, 2017.

[135] 21 U.S.C. 1901-1908 and 8 U.S.C. 1182; U.S. Department of the Treasury, "Treasury Sanctions Chinese Fentanyl Trafficker Jian Zhang," press release, April 27, 2018. See also CRS In Focus IF10909, *International Narcotics Trafficking Sanctions: An Overview*.

similar action against Mexican individuals and entities involved in trafficking heroin and fentanyl to the United States.[136]

What has Mexico Done to Interrupt the Flow of Illicit Opioids into the United States?

The government of Mexico cooperates with the United States on counternarcotics matters, including opioid supply reduction. The government eradicates opium poppy; tracks, seizes, and interdicts opioids and precursor chemicals; dismantles clandestine drug laboratories; and carries out operations against transnational organized crime groups engaged in opioid trafficking and other related crimes. The Mexican government also participates in international efforts to control precursor chemicals, including fentanyl precursors NPP and ANPP.

In 2018, the government of Mexico increased its budget for public security and justice (including antidrug efforts) by 6.2% as compared to 2017, and formed an Office of National Drug Policy within the Attorney General's Office to coordinate federal drug policy.[137] Inaugurated to a six-year term in December 2018, President Andrés Manuel López Obrador has continued cooperation on drug control with the United States. Observers maintain that both governments could find a common interest in combating fentanyl smuggling, but predict that the López Obrador government's proposal to regulate opium cultivation for medicinal purposes could cause friction in bilateral relations.[138]

---

[136] U.S. Department of the Treasury, "Treasury Targets Major Mexican Heroin Trafficking Organization," press release, May 2, 2017; "Treasury Increases Pressure on Mexican Heroin Traffickers," press release, March 6, 2018; U.S. Department of Justice (DOJ), "Justice, Treasury, and State Departments Announce Coordinated Enforcement Efforts Against Cartel Jalisco Nueva Generacion," press release, October 16, 2018; and "'The Drug Llama' Faces Federal Indictment and Mandatory Minimum Sentence for Distributing Fentanyl on Dark Web," press release, September 18, 2018.

[137] U.S. Department of State, *INCSR*, Volume 1, March 2019.

[138] UC San Diego, *U.S.-Mexico Security Cooperation: 2018-2024,* March 2019, https://usmex.ucsd.edu/_files/ Whitepaper_Security_Taskforce_March_26_Covers.pdf; Vanda Felbab-Brown, *AMLO's Security Policy: Creative Ideas, Tough Reality,* Brookings

The Mexican military leads efforts to eradicate illicit drug crops in Mexico, including a reported 29,692 hectares of opium poppy in 2017.[139] Mexican authorities reportedly seized approximately 766.9 kilograms of opium gum[140] in 2017, up from 235 kilograms in 2016.[141] The United States has provided specialized training and equipment to Mexican authorities that contributed to increased fentanyl seizures in 2017 and 2018. Various Mexican agencies have identified and seized fentanyl and fentanyl-laced counterfeit pills with U.S.-funded nonintrusive inspection equipment and canine teams. In September 2018, Mexican law enforcement discovered a production mill used to produce carfentanil (an analogue 100 times more potent than fentanyl).[142]

What has China Done to Interrupt the Flow of Illicit Opioids into the United States?

As discussed, China is a primary source of illicit fentanyl destined for the United States. As of December 1, 2018, China had imposed controls on 170 new psychoactive substances, including 25 fentanyl analogues. It had also imposed controls on two fentanyl precursor chemicals.[143] According to the DEA, U.S. seizure data show that China's implementation of controls on fentanyl analogues has had "an immediate effect on the availability of these drugs in the United States."[144]

Institution, March 2019, https://www.brookings.edu/research/amlos-security-policy-creative-ideas-tough-reality/.

[139] UNODC, "Mexico and UNODC Present Second Opium Poppy Cultivation Survey," November 2018.

[140] Opium gum is a sticky substance that is obtained from the unripe seedpods of the opium poppy.

[141] U.S. Department of State, *INCSR*, Volume 1, March 2019.

[142] Ibid.

[143] "China Lists Another 32 New Psychoactive Substances," *Xinhua*, August 29, 2018, http://www.xinhuanet.com/english/2018-08/29/c_137428313.htm.

[144] Testimony of Daniel D. Baldwin, Section Chief, Office of Global Enforcement, U.S. Drug Enforcement Administration (DEA), U.S. Department of Justice (DOJ), before U.S. Congress, Senate Committee on Homeland Security and Governmental Affairs, Permanent Subcommittee on Investigations, *Combatting the Opioid Crisis: Exploiting Vulnerabilities in International Mail*, 115th Cong., 2nd sess., January 25, 2018, https://

President Xi Jinping said China was willing to go further and control the entire class of fentanyl substances, a move supported by President Trump.[145]

In April 2019, three Chinese government agencies jointly announced that effective May 1, 2019, all fentanyl-related substances will be added to China's "Supplementary List of Controlled Narcotic Drugs and Psychotropic Substances with Non-Medical Use."[146] Li Yuejin, Deputy Director of China's National Narcotics Control Commission, outlined a series of follow-on steps that he said China would take. He said China would issue "guidance on applicable laws for handling criminal cases related to fentanyl substances" and protocols for filing and prosecuting similar cases. Other actions he said China would take include the following:

- investigating suspected illicit fentanyl manufacturing bases;
- scrubbing drug-related content from the Internet;
- "cut[ting] off online communication and transaction channels for criminals";
- pressuring parcel delivery services to require that senders register their real names;
- stepping up inspections of international parcels;
- setting up special teams to conduct criminal investigations focused on manufacturing and trafficking of fentanyl substances and other drugs;

---

www.hsgac.senate.gov/subcommittees/investigations/hearings/combatting-the-opioid-crisis-exploiting- vulnerabilities-in-international-mail.

145 The White House, "President Donald J. Trump's State Visit to China," press release, November 10, 2017; and "Statement from the Press Secretary Regarding the President's Working Dinner with China," December 1, 2018, https://www.whitehouse.gov/briefings-statements/statement-press-secretary-regarding-presidents-working-dinner- china/; and @realDonaldTrump, December 5, 2018, https://twitter.com/realdonaldtrump/status/1070312880095068160.

146 The agencies are the Ministry of Public Security, National Health Commission, and National Medical Products Administration. "SCIO Briefing on Fentanyl-Related Substances Control," April 1, 2019, http://www.china.org.cn/china/2019-04/02/content_74637197.htm.

- strengthening information-sharing and case cooperation with "relevant countries," including the United States, with the goal of dismantling transnational drug smuggling networks; and
- stepping up development of technology for examining and identifying controlled substances.[147]

The DEA welcomed the Chinese government's announcement, saying, "[t]his significant development will eliminate Chinese drug traffickers' ability to alter fentanyl compounds to get around the law."[148] ONDCP noted that China's scheduling decision does not cover all the precursor chemicals used to make fentanyl substances, meaning that they might continue to flow to Mexico where traffickers use them to make fentanyl destined for the United States.[149]

China's postal service, China Post, has an existing agreement with the USPS to provide advanced electronic data (AED) on parcels mailed to the United States.[150] China's government has also cracked down on illicit fentanyl rings in China and assisted DOJ investigations of Chinese nationals suspected of illicit fentanyl manufacturing and distributing.[151]

---

[147] Li identified these pending documents as "Opinions on a Number of Issues Concerning Applicable Laws to Criminal Cases of Fentanyl-Related Substances," "Commutation Table for Dependence of Fentanyl-Related Substances," and "Regulations on Prosecution Standards of Criminal Cases of Fentanyl-Related Substances."

[148] Michael Martina, "U.S. Welcomes China's Expanded Clampdown on Fentanyl," March 31, 2019, Reuters.

[149] Steven Lee Myers and Abby Goodnough, "China Bans All Types of Fentanyl, Cutting Supply of Deadly Drug to U.S. and Fulfilling Pledge to Trump," *The New York Times*, April 1, 2019.

[150] Testimony of Robert Cintron, Vice President, Network Operations, U.S. Postal Service, before U.S. Congress, Senate Committee on Homeland Security and Governmental Affairs, Permanent Subcommittee on Investigations, *Combatting the Opioid Crisis: Exploiting Vulnerabilities in International Mail*, 115th Cong., 2nd sess., January 25, 2018, https://www.hsgac.senate.gov/subcommittees/investigations/hearings/combatting-the-opioid-crisis-exploiting- vulnerabilities-in-international-mail.

[151] See, for example, Department of Justice (DOJ), "Attorney General Sessions Announces New Indictments in International Fentanyl Case," April 27, 2018, https://www.justice.gov/opa/speech/attorney-general-sessions-announces- new-indictments-international-fentanyl-case.

RECENT CONGRESSIONAL ACTION ON THE OPIOID EPIDEMIC

What federal Laws have been Enacted Recently that Address the Opioid Epidemic?

Congress largely has taken a public health approach (i.e., focusing on prevention and treatment) toward addressing the nation's opioid crisis, but recently enacted laws have addressed supply control and other criminal justice issues as well. Three major laws were enacted in the 114th and 115th Congresses that address the opioid epidemic—the Comprehensive Addiction and Recovery Act (CARA, P.L. 114-198); the 21st Century Cures Act (Cures Act; P.L. 114-255); and the SUPPORT for Patients and Communities Act (SUPPORT Act; P.L. 115-271). CARA focused primarily on opioids but also addressed broader drug abuse issues. The Cures Act authorized state opioid grants (in Division A) and included more general substance abuse provisions (in Division B) as part of a larger effort to address health research and treatment. The SUPPORT Act broadly addressed substance use disorder prevention and treatment as well as diversion control through extensive provisions involving law enforcement, public health, and health care financing and coverage.[152] Further, Congress and the Administration provided funds to specifically address opioid abuse in FY2017-FY2019 appropriations.

---

[152] CRS published a series of reports on the SUPPORT Act. See CRS Report R45449, *The SUPPORT for Patients and Communities Act (P.L.115-271): Medicare Provisions*; CRS Report R45423, *Public Health and Other Related Provisions in P.L 115-271, the SUPPORT for Patients and Communities Act*; and CRS Report R45405, *The SUPPORT for Patients and Communities Act (P.L. 115-271): Food and Drug Administration and Controlled Substance Provisions*.

How much FY2019 Funding has Congress Provided DHS, DOJ, and ONDCP to Address the Opioid Epidemic?

Many questions surround the amount of opioid funding appropriated each year. The Consolidated Appropriations Act, 2019 (P.L. 116-6),[153] provided $347.0 million for "comprehensive opioid abuse reduction activities, including as authorized by CARA, and for … programs, which shall address opioid abuse reduction consistent with underlying program authorities"[154] (which includes many of the programs cited above in "Which DOJ grant programs may be used to address the opioid epidemic?"). In FY2019, the DEA received an increase of $77.8 million over FY2018 funding "to help fight drug trafficking, including heroin and fentanyl." The additional DEA funding will also go toward the addition of "at least four new heroin enforcement teams and DEA 360 Strategy programming."[155]

Other opioid-specific funding in FY2019 DOJ, DHS, and ONDCP appropriations includes

- $9.0 million for the Opioid-Affected Youth Initiative;
- $27.0 million for the COPS Program for improving tribal law enforcement, including anti-opioid activities among other purposes (the Tribal Resources Grant Program);
- $32.0 million for anti-heroin task forces (composed of state law enforcement agencies) in areas with high rates of opioid treatment admissions to be used for counter-opioid drug enforcement;
- $24.4 million for CBP for laboratory personnel, port of entry technology, canine personnel, and support staff for opioid detection;

---

[153] For specific line item amounts, see H.Rept. 116-9.

[154] U.S. Congress, House of Representatives, *Making Further Continuing Appropriations for the Department of Homeland Security for Fiscal Year 2019, and for Other Purposes*, Conference Report to Accompany H.J. 31, 116th Cong., February 13, 2019, p. 103.

[155] Ibid., p. 623.

- $44.0 million for Homeland Security Investigations (HSI) for additional personnel (criminal investigators, special agents, intelligence analysts, and support personnel) for domestic and international opioid/fentanyl-related investigations;
- $8.5 million for DHS research and development related to opioids/fentanyl; and
- $3.0 million for ONDCP for Section 103 of CARA - Community-based Coalition Enhancement Grants to Address Local Drug Crises.[156]

Is There an Estimate for How much DOJ and Other Departments Spend on the Opioid Epidemic?

It is problematic, for many reasons, to identify and sum opioid funding. The amounts listed in the section above represent instances where Congress provided opioid-specific funding for agencies and programs within DOJ, DHS, and ONDCP only. It does not include funding for some broader drug programs, such as HIDTA, unless there was a specific appropriation for opioid-related activity. Some programs that can be used for opioid-related purposes—such as the JAG program, which is used for wide-ranging criminal justice purpose areas—are not included in the list. For some programs for which Congress specified opioid-related purposes, the amount appropriated for the program is not necessarily, and often is not, entirely for opioid-related issues.

[156] The goal of the Community-based Coalition Enhancement Grants to Address Local Drug Crises Program is to prevent and reduce the abuse of opioids or methamphetamines and the abuse of prescription medications among youth. For amounts for all programs listed, see U.S. Congress, House of Representatives, *Making Further Continuing Appropriations for the Department of Homeland Security for Fiscal Year 2019, and for Other Purposes*, Conference Report to Accompany H.J. 31, 116th Cong., February 13, 2019.

The Opioid Epidemic and State Criminal Justice Policies

How have Different States Adapted Their Justice Systems to Deal with the Opioid Crisis?

Across the country, states have adapted elements of their criminal justice responses—including police, court, and correctional responses[157]—in a variety of ways due to the opioid epidemic. While this section does not provide a state-by-state analysis, it highlights several examples of how states' justice systems have responded to the opioid crisis. These examples were selected because they are some of the more common state policy approaches to confronting the opioid epidemic.

Many states are increasing law enforcement officer access to naloxone, an opioid overdose reversal drug, in an effort to reduce the number of overdose deaths.[158] Officers receive training on how to identify an opioid overdose and administer naloxone, and they carry the drug so they can respond immediately and effectively to an overdose. As of November 2018, over 2,400 police departments in 42 states reported that they had officers that carry naloxone[159]—this figure more than doubled over two years. In addition, most states that have expanded access to naloxone have also provided immunity to those who possess, dispense, or administer the drug. Generally, immunity entails legal protections (for civilians) from arrest or prosecution and/or civil lawsuits for those who prescribe or dispense naloxone in good faith.[160]

State and local law enforcement coordinate special operations and task forces to combat fentanyl and heroin trafficking in their jurisdictions. In

---

[157] Not all states respond by adapting every component of the criminal justice system.

[158] National Conference of State Legislatures, *Drug Overdose Immunity and Good Samaritan Laws*, June 5, 2017, http://www.ncsl.org/research/civil-and-criminal-justice/drug-overdose-immunity-good-samaritan-laws.aspx.

[159] North Carolina Harm Reduction Coalition (NCHRC), *Law Enforcement Departments Carrying Naloxone*, http://www.nchrc.org/law-enforcement/us-law-enforcement-who-carry-naloxone/.

[160] Some laws also provide disciplinary immunity for medical professionals.

addition to participation in federal initiatives, state and local police and district attorneys lead operations to dismantle trafficking networks in areas plagued by high numbers of opioid overdoses. For example, in southeast Massachusetts[161] the Bristol County District Attorney recently announced the conclusion of a year-long investigation of a "highly organized and complex" fentanyl network that resulted in 11 arrests.[162] This investigation was led by the Bristol Country District Attorney's office and involved several local police agencies, the Massachusetts State Police, and the U.S. Department of Homeland Security.[163]

Another criminal justice adaptation is the enactment of what are known as "Good Samaritan" laws to encourage individuals to seek medical attention (for themselves or others) related to an overdose without fear of arrest or prosecution. In general, these laws prevent criminal prosecution for illegal possession of a controlled substance under specified circumstances. While the laws vary by state as to what offenses and violations are covered, as of June 2017, 40 states and the District of Columbia have some form of Good Samaritan overdose immunity law.[164]

Most states have drug diversion or drug court programs[165] for criminal defendants and offenders with substance abuse issues, including opioid abuse.[166] Some states view drug courts as a tool to address rising opioid abuse and have moved to expand drug court options in the wake of the

---

161 For opioid-related overdose death data in Massachusetts, see Commonwealth of Massachusetts, Executive Office of Health and Human Services, *Current Opioid Statistics*, https://www.mass.gov/lists/current-opioid-statistics.

162 Curt Brown, "'Operation Ghost' nets 11 arrests in New Bedford fentanyl trafficking ring," *South Coast Today*, April 30, 2019.

163 Ibid.

164 National Conference of State Legislatures, *Drug Overdose Immunity and Good Samaritan Laws*, June 5, 2017, http://www.ncsl.org/research/civil-and-criminal-justice/drug-overdose-immunity-good-samaritan-laws.aspx.

165 Some specialized court programs are designed to divert certain defendants and offenders away from traditional criminal justice sanctions such as incarceration while reducing overall costs and helping these defendants and offenders with substance abuse issues. Drug court programs may exist at various points in the justice system, but they are often employed post-arrest as an alternative to traditional criminal justice processing. For more information, see CRS Report R44467, *Federal Support for Drug Courts: In Brief.*

166 National Governors Association, *States Expand Opioid Addiction Treatment in Drug Courts, Corrections*, April 11, 2017, https://www.nga.org/cms/news/2017/states-expand-opioid-addiction-treatment. For more information, see CRS Report R44467, *Federal Support for Drug Courts: In Brief.*

opioid epidemic. Over the last several years, the National Governors Association has sponsored various activities to assist states in combatting the opioid epidemic, including learning labs to develop best practices for dealing with opioid abuse treatment for justice-involved populations—such as the expansion of opioid addiction treatment in drug courts.[167] In November 2017, the President's Commission on Combating Drug Addiction and the Opioid Crisis stated that DOJ should urge states to establish drug courts in every county.[168]

In recent years, several states have also enacted legislation increasing access to medication- assisted treatment (MAT) for drug-addicted offenders who are incarcerated or have recently been released.[169] In March 2019, SAMHSA released guidance to state governments on increasing the availability of MAT in criminal justice settings.[170]

---

[167] National Governors Association, *States Expand Opioid Addiction Treatment in Drug Courts, Corrections*, April 11, 2017, https://www.nga.org/cms/news/2017/states-expand-opioid-addiction-treatment; and *Drug Policy*, https://www.nga.org/center/issues/drug-policy/.

[168] The President's Commission on Combating Drug Addiction and the Opioid Crisis, *Final Report*, November 1, 2017, p. 10.

[169] National Conference of State Legislatures, *American Epidemic: Overdose on Opioids*, State Legislatures Magazine, April 2016, http://www.ncsl.org/bookstore/state-legislatures-magazine/overdosed-on-opioids.aspx.

[170] U.S. Department of Health and Human Services (HHS), Substance Abuse and Mental Health Services Administration (SAMHSA), *Medication-Assisted Treatment (MAT) in the Criminal Justice System: Brief Guidance to the States*, March 2019, https://store.samhsa.gov/product/Medication-Assisted-Treatment-MAT-in-the-Criminal- Justice-System-Brief-Guidance-to-the-States/PEP19-MATBRIEFCJS.

In: Key Congressional Reports for June 2019 ISBN: 978-1-53616-665-1
Editor: Amada A. Byrd

Chapter 6

SOCIAL SECURITY: WHAT WOULD HAPPEN IF THE TRUST FUNDS RAN OUT? (UPDATED)*

Barry F. Huston and William R. Morton

SUMMARY

Social Security's receipts and expenditures are accounted for through two federal trust funds: the Federal Old-Age and Survivors Insurance (OASI) Trust Fund and the Federal Disability Insurance (DI) Trust Fund. Under their intermediate assumptions and under current law, the Social Security trustees project that the DI trust fund will become depleted in 2052 and the OASI trust fund will become depleted in 2034. Although the two funds are legally separate, they are often considered in combination. The trustees project that the combined Social Security trust funds will become depleted in 2035. At that point, the combined trust funds would become *insolvent*, because incoming tax revenue would be sufficient to pay only about 80% of scheduled benefits.

---

* This is an edited, reformatted and augmented version of Congressional Research Service Publication No. RL33514, Updated June 12, 2019.

If a trust fund became depleted and current receipts were insufficient to cover current expenditures, there would be a conflict between two federal laws. Under the Social Security Act, beneficiaries would still be legally entitled to their full scheduled benefits. However, the Antideficiency Act prohibits government spending in excess of available funds, so the Social Security Administration (SSA) would not have legal authority to pay full Social Security benefits on time.

It is unclear what specific actions SSA would take if a trust fund were insolvent. After depletion, the trust funds would continue to receive tax revenues, from which a majority of scheduled benefits could be paid. One option would be to pay full benefits on a delayed schedule; another would be to make timely but reduced payments. Social Security beneficiaries would remain legally entitled to full, timely benefits and could take legal action to claim the balance of their benefits.

Maintaining financial balance after trust fund insolvency would require substantial reductions in Social Security benefits, substantial increases in tax revenues, or some combination of the two. The trustees project that following depletion of the combined funds in 2035, Congress could restore balance by reducing scheduled benefits by about 20%; the required reduction would grow gradually to 25% by 2093. An alternative could be for Congress to raise the Social Security payroll tax rate from 12.4% to 15.60% following depletion in 2035, then gradually increase it to 16.50% by 2093.

Trust-fund insolvency could be avoided if expenditures were reduced or receipts increased sufficiently. The sooner Congress acts to adjust Social Security policy, the less abrupt the changes would need to be, because they could be spread over a longer period and would therefore affect a larger number of workers and beneficiaries. Even if changes were not implemented immediately, enacting them sooner would give workers and beneficiaries more time to plan and adjust their work and savings behavior.

INTRODUCTION

Each year when the Social Security trustees release their annual report, attention is focused on the projection of the year that the Social Security trust funds will become *depleted*, that is, the year in which the trust funds' investment holdings in U.S. Treasury securities fall to zero.[1] In their 2019

[1] The Social Security Board of Trustees presents an annual report to Congress on the current and projected financial status of the Social Security trust funds (see 42 U.S.C. §401[c]). The

report, the trustees project that, under their intermediate assumptions and under current law, the Federal Disability Insurance (DI) Trust Fund will become depleted in 2052 and the Federal Old-Age and Survivors Insurance (OASI) Trust Fund will do so in 2034.[2] Although the two funds are legally separate, they are often described in combination. The trustees project that the combined Old-Age, Survivors, Disability Insurance (OASDI) trust funds will become depleted in 2035.

Some Americans may believe that if the trust funds were depleted, Social Security would be unable to pay benefits at all. In fact, in 2035, the first year of projected depletion of the combined Social Security trust funds, the program is projected to have enough tax revenues to pay about 80% of scheduled benefits; that percentage would decline to 75% by the end of the 75-year projection period in 2093.[3] Thus, although the trust funds would be *insolvent* upon depletion, because they would be unable to cover 100% of expenditures with incoming tax revenues, they would not be "completely broke" and unable to pay *any* benefits.

Although benefits would be paid in some form, it is unclear how the necessary reductions would be implemented, because the Social Security Act does not specify what would happen to benefits if a trust fund became insolvent. One option would be to pay full benefits on a delayed schedule; another would be to make timely but reduced payments.

This chapter explains what the Social Security trust funds are and how they work. It describes the historical operations of the trust funds and the Social Security trustees' projections of future operations. It explains what

---

board is composed of six members: the Secretary of the Treasury, who is the Managing Trustee; the Secretary of Labor; the Secretary of Health and Human Services; the Commissioner of Social Security; and two public representatives, who are nominated by the President for a term of four years and subject to confirmation by the Senate. The trustees specify the assumptions about future demographic and economic trends used in the projections; however, the Social Security Administration's (SSA) Office of the Chief Actuary (OCACT) advises the trustees on the assumptions as well as develops and runs the computer models that produce the forecasts.

[2] The Board of Trustees, Federal Old-Age and Survivors Insurance and Federal Disability Insurance Trust Funds, The 2019 Annual Report of the Board of Trustees of the Federal Old-Age and Survivors Insurance and Federal Disability Insurance Trust Funds, April 25, 2019, Table IV.B4, https://www.ssa.gov/OACT/TR/2019/tr2019.pdf (hereinafter "2019 Social Security Trustees Report").

[3] Ibid., Table IV.B4.

could happen if Congress allowed the trust funds to run out. It also analyzes two scenarios that assume Congress waits until the moment of insolvency to act, showing the magnitude of benefit cuts or tax increases needed and how such changes would affect beneficiaries.

BACKGROUND ON SOCIAL SECURITY

Old-Age, Survivors, and Disability Insurance, commonly known as Social Security, is a work-related social insurance program authorized under Title II of the Social Security Act that provides monthly cash benefits to retired or disabled workers and their eligible dependents and to eligible survivors of deceased insured workers.[4] Workers obtain insurance protection by working for a sufficient number of years in jobs covered by Social Security. A worker's job is considered *covered* if the earnings derived from that job are subject to Social Security taxes and thus are creditable for program purposes. In 2019, an estimated 177 million people (or about 93% of all workers) will work in paid employment or self-employment covered by Social Security.[5]

Social Security benefits are based on a worker's career-average earnings in jobs covered by Social Security and designed to replace a portion of the income lost to a family due to the worker's retirement, disability, or death. In April 2019, the Social Security Administration (SSA) authorized benefit payments for 63.4 million beneficiaries, including 44.2 million retired workers, 8.5 million disabled workers, 4.7 million dependents of retired or disabled workers, and 6.0 million survivors of deceased insured workers.[6] The average benefit payment issued that month was $1,468 for retired workers, $1,235 for disabled

[4] 42 U.S.C. §§401 et seq.

[5] SSA, OCACT, *Fact Sheet on the Old-Age, Survivors, and Disability Insurance Program*, December 31, 2018, https://www.ssa.gov/oact/FACTS/index.html.

[6] SSA, OCACT, "Benefits Paid By Type Of Beneficiary," https://www.ssa.gov/oact/ProgData/icp.html.

workers, $624 for dependents of retired or disabled workers, and $1,193 for survivors for deceased insured workers.[7]

THE SOCIAL SECURITY TRUST FUNDS

How the Trust Funds Work[8]

Social Security's receipts and expenditures are accounted for through two legally distinct federal trust funds: the OASI trust fund and the DI trust fund. In the federal accounting structure, a *trust fund* is an accounting mechanism used by the Department of the Treasury to track and report receipts dedicated for spending on specific purposes, as well as expenditures made to its beneficiaries that are financed by those receipts, in accordance with the terms of a statute that designates the fund as a trust fund.[9] The OASI trust fund records receipts and expenditures associated with retired workers, their dependents, and survivors of deceased insured workers, while the DI trust fund records receipts and expenditures associated with disabled workers and their dependents. The OASI and DI trust funds operate separately but are closely linked.[10] Several times in the past, Congress has authorized the reallocation of the Social Security payroll tax rate to equalize the financial conditions of the two trust funds. In part because of those experiences, analysts often treat the two funds collectively on a hypothetical basis as the combined OASDI trust funds.

The Social Security trust funds, like most federal trust funds, have different attributes than trust funds in the private sector. The Government Accountability Office (GAO) notes the following:

---

[7] Ibid.

[8] CRS Report RL33028, Social Security: The Trust Funds.

[9] An account of the U.S. Treasury is designated as a trust fund by the Office of Management and Budget (OMB), in consultation with the Department of the Treasury, if the fund's authorizing legislation makes such a designation and if the fund's receipts are earmarked for spending on specific purposes or programs. Section 201 of the Social Security Act (42 U.S.C. §401) authorizes the Federal Old-Age and Survivors Insurance (OASI) Trust Fund and the Federal Disability Insurance (DI) Trust Fund and designates them as trust funds.

[10] Under current law, the OASI and DI trust funds may not borrow from one another.

In the federal budget the meaning of the term "trust" differs significantly from its private sector usage. In the private sector, a person creates a private trust fund using his or her own assets to benefit a stated individual(s). The creator of the trust names a trustee who has a fiduciary responsibility to manage the designated assets in accordance with the stipulations of the trust. In the federal sector, the Congress creates a federal trust fund in law and designates a funding source to benefit stated groups or individuals. However, in contrast to a private trust fund, the federal government does not have a fiduciary responsibility to the trust beneficiaries, and it can raise or lower future trust fund collections and payments or change the purposes for which the collections are used by changing existing laws. Moreover, the federal government has custody and control of the funds as well as the earnings of most federal trust funds.[11]

Trust Fund Receipts

The trust funds' primary source of revenue is the Social Security payroll tax, but they also receive income from federal income taxes on benefits and from interest on the funds' investment holdings. The payroll tax consists of a 12.40% total tax on wages and self-employment income up to the taxable maximum, which in 2019 is $132,900 and generally increases annually with average earnings growth in the economy.[12] Of the 12.40% total, 10.03% is credited to the OASI trust fund and 2.37% to the DI trust fund.[13] Some Social Security benefits paid to people with incomes above a certain threshold are subject to federal income tax.[14] Most of the resulting revenue is credited to the Social Security trust funds, and some goes to Medicare's Hospital Insurance (HI) trust fund.[15] In 2018, the combined trust funds' total receipts were $1,003.4 billion, with 88.2%

---

[11] .S. Government Accountability Office (GAO), *Federal Trust and Other Earmarked Funds: Answers to Frequently Asked Questions*, GAO-01-199SP, January 1, 2001, p. 7, https://www.gao.gov/products/GAO-01-199SP.

[12] 42 U.S.C. §430 and 26 U.S.C. §§1401, 3101, and 3111. See SSA, OCACT, "Contribution and Benefit Base," https://www.ssa.gov/oact/cola/cbb.html.

[13] 42 U.S.C. §401(a) and 401(b). Both the total tax rate and the allocation of it between the OASI and DI trust funds have changed many times; for historical rates, see SSA, OCACT, "Social Security Taxes Rates," https://www.ssa.gov/ oact/progdata/oasdiRates.html.

[14] CRS Report RL32552, Social Security: Calculation and History of Taxing Benefits.

[15] CRS Report R43122, Medicare Financial Status: In Brief.

from payroll taxes, 8.3% from interest income, and 3.5% from income taxes on benefits (see *Appendix A*).[16]

Trust Fund Expenditures

In 2018, the combined trust funds' total expenditures were $1,000.2 billion, with 98.8% for benefit payments and 0.7% for administrative expenses (see *Appendix A*). The remaining 0.5% was transferred to the Railroad Retirement Board (RRB) as part of a financial interchange with the RRB. This annual exchange of funds places the Social Security trust funds in the same financial position in which they would have been if railroad service had been covered by Social Security.

Annual Surpluses and Deficits

In years when Social Security's total receipts, including interest, exceed expenditures, then the trust funds have an *annual surplus*. By law, that surplus is invested in special-issue U.S. Treasury securities (i.e., nonmarketable government bonds), which are backed by the full faith and credit of the federal government. In other words, Social Security's cash surpluses are borrowed by the General Fund of the U.S. Treasury. The Treasury, in turn, incurs an obligation to repay the bonds with interest. These bonds are assets to the Social Security program but liabilities to the rest of the government. In 2018, the combined trust funds generated an annual surplus of $3.1 billion ($1,003.4 billion in total receipts *minus* $1,000.2 billion in total expenditures; see *Appendix A*).

When the trust funds spend more than they receive in taxes and interest, they have an *annual deficit,* which requires Social Security to redeem bonds accumulated in previous years. The Department of the Treasury pays benefits with cash from general revenues and writes down an equivalent amount of the trust fund's bond holdings.[17] In their latest

---

[16] SSA, OCACT, "Trust Fund Data," https://www.ssa.gov/oact/ProgData/funds.html. A very small amount of the combined trust funds total receipts (about 0.002%) were transfers from the General Fund of the U.S. Treasury, which occurred for several different reasons.

[17] See David Pattison, "Social Security Trust Fund Cash Flows and Reserves," *Social Security Bulletin*, vol. 75, no. 1 (February 2015), https://www.ssa.gov/policy/docs/ssb/v75 n1/index. html.

report, the Social Security trustees project that total expenditures for the combined trust funds will exceed total receipts in 2020, resulting in an annual deficit for the first time since 1982.[18]

Cash-Flow Surpluses and Deficits

An alternative measure of the trust funds' finances is given by the *cash-flow* balance. That measure does not consider interest income, so the trust funds run a *cash-flow surplus* when tax revenues exceed expenditures, and they run a *cash-flow deficit* when they spend more than they receive in taxes.

Total receipts for the combined trust funds in 2018 were $1,003.4 billion, with $920.1 billion in noninterest income (i.e., payroll taxes and income taxes on benefits) and $83.3 billion in interest income (see *Appendix A*). Because total expenditures for the combined trust funds in 2018 were $1,000.2 billion, there was a combined cash-flow deficit in 2018 of $80.1 billion ($1,000.2 billion in total expenditures *minus* $920.1 billion in noninterest income).

Trust Fund Balances

The *balance* of a trust fund is the accumulation of excess receipts over expenditures (i.e., the sum of annual surpluses *less* annual deficits). A positive balance denotes the total amount of the trust fund's investment holdings in U.S. government bonds (also known as *asset reserves*). Annual surpluses add to a trust fund's balance while annual deficits reduce it. The annual surplus of $3.1 billion in 2018 increased the trust funds' combined balance from $2,891 billion at the end of 2017 to $2,894 billion at the end of 2018 (see *Appendix A*).

Trust Fund Solvency

If the trust funds are not able to pay all of current expenditures out of current tax revenues and accumulated trust fund assets, they are *insolvent*. Insolvency means that Social Security's trust funds are unable to pay

---

[18] 2019 Social Security Trustees Report, p. 2 and Table VI.G8 (Supplemental Single-Year Table).

benefits in full and on time. It does *not* mean that Social Security will be "completely broke" and unable to pay any benefits.

Historical Trust Fund Operations

The OASI trust fund was created by the Social Security Act Amendments of 1939 (P.L. 76-379) and superseded the Old-Age Reserve Account established by the original Social Security Act in 1935 (P.L. 74-271).[19] The DI trust fund was established as part of the Social Security Amendments of 1956 (P.L. 84-880).[20] Neither of the Social Security trust funds has ever become insolvent. The trust funds have existed on a hypothetical combined basis since the DI fund was first credited with receipts and debited for expenditures in 1957.

Surpluses and Deficits

The trust funds have run *annual surpluses* in most years. Except for the first decades of the program and a few years beginning in the late 1960s, these annual surpluses were typically small relative to the size of the trust funds' expenditures. Beginning in 1975, the combined trust funds ran annual deficits. The trust funds made up the difference between receipts and expenditures during these years by redeeming some of the bonds accumulated in earlier years. In other words, in those years, the Social Security trust funds received net transfers from the Treasury's General Fund.

The aging of the baby-boom population and the recent recession and subsequent weak economy have resulted in higher expenditures and lower tax revenues for Social Security. Since 2010, the combined trust funds

---

[19] The OASI trust fund became effective on January 1, 1940. For more information on the origins of the OASI trust fund and the Old-Age Reserve Account, see Board of Trustees of the Federal Old-Age and Survivors Insurance Trust Fund, *First Report of the Board of Trustees of the Federal Old-Age and Survivors Insurance Trust Fund*, January 3, 1941, https://www.ssa.gov/oact/tr/historical/1941TR.html.

[20] The DI trust fund was established on August 1, 1956. For more information on the origins of the DI Trust Fund, see CRS Report R43318, *The Social Security Disability Insurance (DI) Trust Fund: Background and Current Status.*

have run cash-flow deficits (*Figure 1*), which are projected to continue indefinitely under current law.

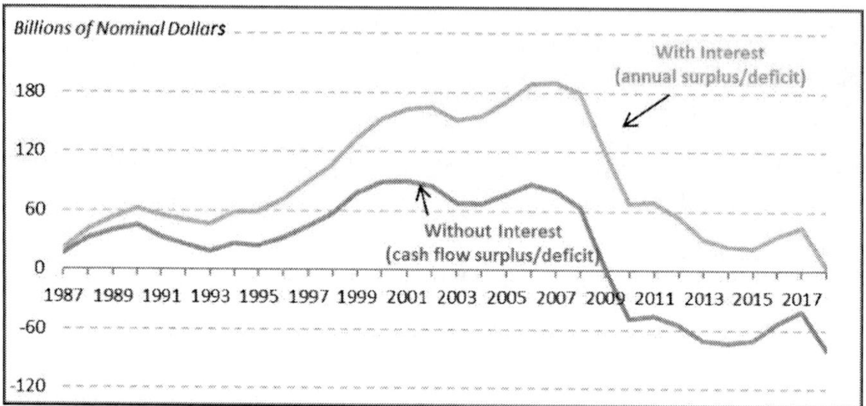

Source: Congressional Research Service (CRS), based on data from the Social Security Administration (SSA), Office of the Chief Actuary (OCACT), "Social Security Trust Fund Data," https://www.ssa.gov/oact/STATS/ table4a3.html.

Figure 1. Annual Net Change in the Balance of the Combined Social Security Trust Funds, With and Without Interest Income, 1987-2018.

However, because interest income has exceeded the *cash-flow deficit*, the combined trust funds have continued to run annual surpluses, which averaged about 5% of total expenditures from 2010 through 2018.[21] Cash-flow deficits do not affect Social Security directly. However, if the non-Social Security portion of the federal budget is in deficit, redemption of trust fund bonds puts additional pressure on the overall federal budget.

Near-Insolvency of the OASI Trust Fund in the Early 1980s

In the early 1980s, a solvency crisis loomed for the OASI trust fund. The 1982 Social Security Trustees Report projected that in the absence of legislative changes, the OASI trust fund would become insolvent by July 1983.[22] To relieve the pressure on the OASI trust fund temporarily,

---

[21] SSA, OCACT, "Social Security Trust Fund Data," https://www.ssa.gov/oact/ProgData/ funds.html.

[22] U.S. Congress, House Committee on Ways and Means, The 1982 Annual Report of the Board of Trustees of the Federal Old-Age and Survivors Insurance and Federal Disability

Congress permitted the fund to borrow from the DI and HI trust funds through the end of 1982.[23] On November 5, 1982, the Department of the Treasury announced that the balance of the OASI trust fund had fallen to zero, and that the U.S. Treasury would be unable to redeem the amount of bonds necessary to cover the OASI benefit checks that had been delivered on November 3.[24] To cover the shortfall, the Secretary of the Treasury authorized a $581 million loan from the DI trust fund to the OASI trust fund. Additional loans from the DI and HI trust funds to the OASI trust fund were made before the temporary interfund borrowing authority expired.

This measure gave policymakers time to develop a more sustainable solution to Social Security's solvency problem. The Social Security Amendments of 1983 (P.L. 98-21) increased Social Security income and reduced spending. As a result, the combined trust funds ran significant surpluses, which on average exceeded a quarter of expenditures from 1987 to 2009. The 1982 loans from the DI and HI trust funds to the OASI trust fund were repaid, with interest, by the end of April 1986.[25]

Recent Near-Insolvency of the DI Trust Fund[26]

In their annual reports for 2012 through 2015, the trustees projected that the DI trust fund would be depleted in late 2016 (see *Appendix B*). At the end of 2015, the balance of the DI trust fund was $32.3 billion, down from $60.2 billion at the start of the year.[27] The declining solvency of the

---

Insurance Trust Funds, 97th Cong., 2nd sess., April 1, 1982, H.Doc. 97-163 (Washington: GPO, 1982), p. 2, https://www.ssa.gov/oact/tr/historical/1982TR.pdf (hereinafter "1982 Social Security Trustees Report").

[23] P.L. 97-123.

[24] Edward Cowan, "Leaders of Both Parties Facing Tough Choices on Social Security Problems," *The New York Times*, November 7, 1982, http://www.nytimes.com/ 1982/11/07/us/leaders-of-both-parties-facing-tough-choices-on-socialsecurity-problems. html. See also see Bruce D. Schobel, "Interfund Borrowing Under the Social Security Act," *Social Security Bulletin*, vol. 46, no. 9 (September 1983), https://www. ssa.gov/ policy/docs/ssb/v46n9/.

[25] SSA, "Research Note #4: Inter-Fund Borrowing Among the Trust Funds," http://www.ssa. gov/history/ interfundnote.html.

[26] CRS Report R43318, *The Social Security Disability Insurance (DI) Trust Fund: Background and Current Status*.

[27] SSA, OCACT, "Time Series for Selected Financial Items," https://www.ssa.gov/oact/Prog Data/tsOps.html.

DI trust fund was the result of an imbalance between the fund's receipts and expenditures. Between 1995 and 2015, tax revenues to the DI trust fund were relatively flat as a percentage of taxable payroll, whereas expenditures as a share of taxable payroll grew markedly.[28] The increase in expenditures stemmed largely from the growth in the number of beneficiaries in the program. During that period, the number of disabled-worker beneficiaries increased by 113%, from nearly 4.2 million to more than 8.9 million.[29]

On November 2, 2015, President Barack Obama signed into law the Bipartisan Budget Act of 2015 (BBA 2015; P.L. 114-74). Among other provisions, the BBA 2015 authorized a temporary reallocation of the payroll tax rate between the OASI and DI trust funds to provide DI with a larger share for 2016 through 2018. Specifically, the DI trust fund's share of the combined tax rate increased by 0.57 percentage points at the beginning of 2016, from 1.80% to 2.37%. Because the BBA 2015 did not change the combined payroll tax rate of 12.40%, the portion of the tax rate allocated to OASI decreased by a corresponding amount. This means that OASI's share of the combined tax rate declined by 0.57 percentage points at the start of 2016, from 10.60% to 10.03%. For 2019 and later, the shares allocated to the DI and OASI trust funds are scheduled to return to their 2015 levels: 1.80% to the DI trust fund and 10.60% to the OASI trust fund.

Social Security Financial Projections

This chapter focuses on the trustees' "intermediate" Social Security projections, which reflect their "best estimates" of future demographic and economic trends.[30] Under that set of assumptions, the DI Trust Fund is

---

[28] *Taxable payroll* is the total amount of earnings in the economy that is subject to Social Security payroll taxes (with some adjustments).

[29] SSA, OCACT, "Benefits Paid by Type of Beneficiary," https://www.ssa.gov/oact/ProgData/icp.html.

[30] To estimate the future financial status of the trust funds, the Social Security trustees produce short-range and long-range actuarial projections under three sets of economic and demographic assumptions: intermediate, low-cost, and high-cost. Intermediate assumptions represent the trustees' best estimate of the financial condition of the trust funds in the future.

depleted in 2052 and the OASI Trust Fund is depleted in 2034.[31] Considered on a hypothetical combined basis, the trust funds would become insolvent in 2035. However, the trustees' projections—like all long-term projections—are uncertain. They estimate that there is a 10% chance that the combined trust funds would become insolvent in 2032 or earlier and a 10% chance that insolvency would occur in 2040 or later.[32] Using somewhat different assumptions and projection methods, the Congressional Budget Office (CBO) projects that the combined trust funds will become insolvent in 2031.[33]

Even after insolvency, the trust funds will continue to receive income from payroll taxes and income taxes on benefits that will allow some benefits to be paid. The trustees project that, under their intermediate assumptions, tax income would be sufficient to cover about 80% of scheduled benefits following insolvency of the combined trust funds in 2035, declining to 75% in 2093.[34]

Trust Fund Ratio

To put the trust fund balance in context, analysts commonly consider the *trust fund ratio*: the balance in the trust funds at the beginning of a year divided by projected expenditures for that year. The trust fund ratio thus represents the proportion of a year's cost that could be paid solely with the reserves at the beginning of the year. The ratio for the combined trust funds peaked at 358% in 2008 (*Figure 2*). The combined trust fund ratio declined

---

The low-cost and high-cost sets of assumptions, on the other hand, depict extraordinarily favorable (low-cost) or unfavorable (high-cost) possibilities for the trust funds' future solvency. According to the trustees, "actual future costs are unlikely to be as extreme as those portrayed by the low-cost and high-cost projections" (2019 Social Security Trustees Report, p. 17). Unless otherwise specified, projections cited in this report are based on the trustees' intermediate assumptions.

[31] 2019 Social Security Trustees Report, Table IV.B4.

[32] Ibid., Table VI.E1.

[33] U.S. Congressional Budget Office (CBO), *The 2018 Long-Term Budget Outlook*, June 26, 2018, p. 17, https://www.cbo.gov/system/files/2018-06/53919-2018ltbo.pdf. Under its 2018 extended baseline and under current law, CBO projects that the DI trust fund will become depleted in FY2025, and the OASI trust fund will become depleted in calendar year 2032. (Newer projections for the OASI and combined trust funds have not been released by CBO as of the date of this report.)

[34] 2019 Social Security Trustees Report, Table IV.B4.

to 289% in 2018 and is continuing to fall. By definition, the ratio will reach zero when the trust funds become depleted.

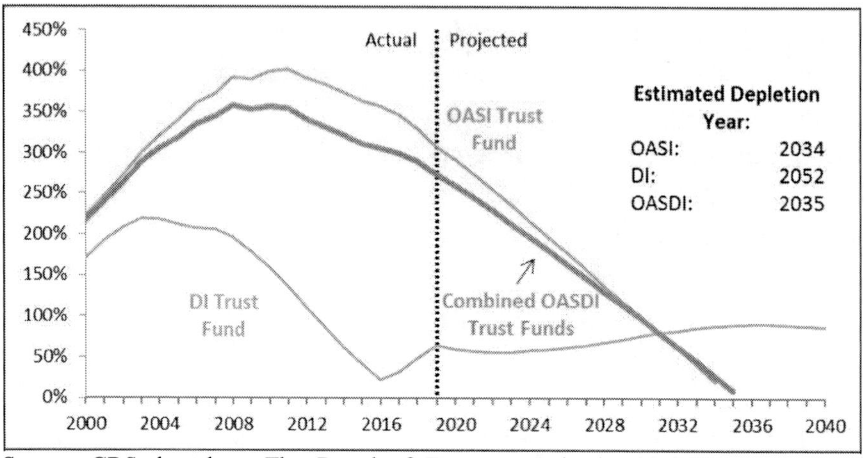

Source: CRS, based on The Board of Trustees, Federal Old-Age and Survivors Insurance and Federal Disability Insurance Trust Funds, The 2019 Annual Report of the Board of Trustees of the Federal Old-Age and Survivors Insurance and Federal Disability Insurance Trust Funds., April 25, 2019, Table IV.B4 (Supplemental Single-Year Table), https://www.ssa.gov/oact/TR/2019/lrIndex.html (hereinafter "2019 Social Security Trustees Report").

Notes: OASI = Old-Age and Survivors Insurance. DI = Disability Insurance. OASDI = Old-Age, Survivors, and Disability Insurance. Projections are based on the trustees' 2019 intermediate assumptions.

Figure 2. Actual and Projected Trust Fund Ratios, by Trust Fund, 2000-2040. (Trust fund assets at the beginning of the year as a share of annual expenditures).

LEGAL BACKGROUND ON TRUST FUND INSOLVENCY

The Antideficiency Act

The Social Security Act specifies that benefit payments shall be made *only* from the trust funds (i.e., only from their accumulated bond holdings).[35] Another law, the Antideficiency Act, prohibits government spending in excess of available funds.[36] Consequently, if the Social Security trust funds become insolvent—that is, if current tax receipts and accumulated assets are not sufficient to pay the benefits to which people are entitled—the law effectively prohibits full Social Security benefits from being paid on time.

Legal Entitlement to Social Security Benefits

The Social Security Act states that every individual who meets program eligibility requirements is entitled to benefits.[37] Social Security is an *entitlement program*, which means that the federal government is legally obligated to pay Social Security benefits to all those who are eligible for them as set forth in the statute.[38] If the federal government fails to pay the benefits stipulated by law, beneficiaries could take legal action. Insolvency would not relieve the government of its obligation to provide benefits.

What Happens to Benefits in the Case of Insolvency?

The Antideficiency Act prohibits government agencies from paying for benefits, goods, or services beyond the limit authorized in law for such payments. The authorized limit in law for Social Security benefits is the balance of the trust fund. The Social Security Act does not stipulate what would happen to benefit payments if the trust funds ran out. As a result, either full benefit checks may be paid on a delayed schedule or reduced

---

[35] 42 U.S.C. §401(h).

[36] 31 U.S.C. §1341.

[37] 42 U.S.C. §§402 and 423.

[38] See 2 U.S.C. §622 for the definition of *entitlement authority*. Congress retains the right to modify provisions of the Social Security Act at any time, which could affect the benefits current and future beneficiaries may receive (see 42 U.S.C. §1304). For more information, see nondistributable CRS Report RL32822, *Social Security Reform: Legal Analysis of Social Security Benefit Entitlement Issues* (available upon request to congressional clients).

benefits would be paid on time.[39] In either case, total payable benefits would be lower than scheduled benefits.

Table 1. Current Social Security Benefit Payment Schedule

Benefits Paid On	Birth Date of Worker on Whose Record Benefits Are Paid
Third of every month	Any birth date for: (1) Social Security beneficiaries who also receive Supplemental Security Income benefits or who reside in a foreign country, and (2) Most beneficiaries who began to receive benefits prior to June 1997.
Second Wednesday	1st to 10th day of the month
Third Wednesday	11th to 20th day of the month.
Fourth Wednesday	21st to 31st day of the month

Source: Congressional Research Service (CRS), based on 20 C.F.R. §404.1807 and Social Security Administration (SSA), Office of the Chief Actuary (OCACT), "Cyclical Payment of Social Security Benefits," http://ssa.gov/OACT/ProgData/cyclicalpay.html.

Note: For beneficiaries scheduled to receive payments on the third of the month, benefits may be paid earlier if the third is on a weekend or holiday.

To see how a delay could affect beneficiaries, consider the current Social Security benefit payment schedule, shown in *Table 1*. (This schedule may be changed at the discretion of the Commissioner of Social Security.)[40]

New beneficiaries' payment dates are generally based on their day of birth—for example, if a retired worker was born on the first of the month (e.g., June 1), his or her benefit payment is made on the second Wednesday in the month.[41]

---

[39] The 1982 Trustees Report, which projected impending trust fund insolvency, stated that unless legislative changes were made, "inability to pay some benefits *on time* would result" (1982 Social Security Trustees Report, p. 2 [emphasis added]). That language suggests that after insolvency, full benefit payments would have been made on a delayed schedule. The 2019 report uses more neutral language, stating that after insolvency, the trust funds would be "unable to pay scheduled benefits in full on a timely basis" (2019 Social Security Trustees Report, p. 5).

[40] 20 C.F.R. §404.1807. For the payment schedule rationale, see SSA, "Cycling Payment of Social Security," 62 *Federal Register* 6114, February 11, 1997, https://www.gpo.gov/fdsys/pkg/FR-1997-02-11/pdf/97-3205.pdf.

[41] For beneficiaries who receive Social Security benefits based on another person's work record (e.g., spousal benefits), their payment date depends on the birth date of the worker on whose

If trust fund insolvency caused delays in the payment schedule, benefit payments could be made in the usual order—first to those who receive benefits on the third of the month, then to those on the second Wednesday of the month, and so on, until the remainder of the trust funds' balance reached zero. At that point, no benefits could be paid until more tax receipts were credited to the trust funds. Then benefit payments could be picked up where they left off when the trust funds ran out. This cycle could continue indefinitely. The timing of these payments would be unpredictable.

WHAT IF CONGRESS WAITS TO ACT?

There are many options to restore Social Security solvency, which could be combined or targeted in a variety of ways. For example, Congress could decrease Social Security benefits. Benefit cuts could be applied proportionately to all beneficiaries or structured to protect certain people, such as disabled or low-income beneficiaries. Congress could also increase Social Security's income by raising payroll or other taxes or by transferring funds from the Treasury's general fund. Payroll tax increases could be applied proportionately to all workers or targeted to certain workers, such as those who earn more than the taxable maximum ($132,900 in 2019).

The next section presents two policy options that could be implemented after the trust funds' combined balance fell to zero to ensure a balanced system in later years:

- the *benefit cut scenario*, under which benefits would be cut across the board; and
- the *tax increase scenario*, under which the payroll tax rate would increase.

---

record they receive benefits. The current benefit payment schedule was first implemented for new beneficiaries in May 1997.

Both scenarios assume that current law would remain in place until the combined trust funds became insolvent. If changes were made sooner, they could be smaller, since the burden of lower benefits or higher taxes would be shared by more beneficiaries or workers over a longer period.[42] Either scenario would essentially convert Social Security to a pure pay-as-you-go system, in which income and outgo are equal on an annual basis and there are no trust fund assets. These scenarios are only two of a wide range of possibilities. When Congress last addressed Social Security's solvency in 1983, lawmakers employed a combination of tax increases and benefit reductions to improve the financial condition of the combined trust funds.

Benefit Cut Scenario

Size of Benefit Cuts

If the trust funds were allowed to run out, Congress could eliminate annual cash-flow deficits by cutting benefits so that spending equals tax income on an annual basis. According to the trustees, achieving annual balance would require benefit cuts of 20% in 2035, the first year of insolvency, rising to 25% by 2093.[43] To maintain balance after 2093, the Social Security trustees project that larger benefit reductions would be needed, because people would continue to live longer and therefore collect benefits for longer periods.

Figure 3 shows the percentage of scheduled benefits that are payable each year with scheduled revenues. One way to understand how such a reduction would affect beneficiaries is to examine the effect on projected replacement rates and real benefit amounts for hypothetical workers.

---

[42] The trustees estimate that 75-year solvency could be restored through (1) an immediate payroll tax increase of 2.70 percentage points (from the current 12.40% to 15.10%), (2) a benefit reduction of 17% for all current and future beneficiaries, (3) a benefit reduction of 20% for only those who become initially eligible for benefits in 2019 or later, or (4) some combination of those approaches. If Congress waited until 2035 to act, the trustees estimate that maintaining solvency over the 75-year projection period would require (1) a payroll tax increase of 3.65 percentage points (from the current 12.40% to 16.05%) starting in 2035, (2) a reduction in scheduled benefits of 23% starting in 2035, or (3) some combination of those approaches. See 2019 Social Security Trustees Report, pp. 4-5.

[43] 2019 Social Security Trustees Report, Table IV.B4.

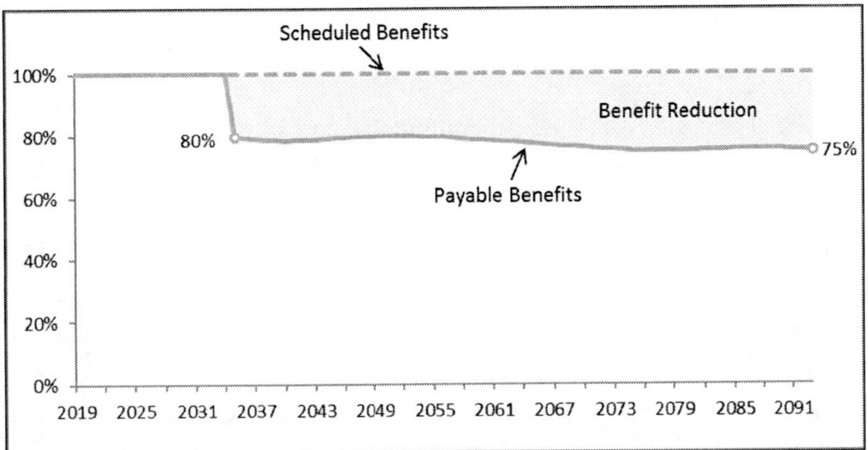

Source: CRS, based on an OCACT memorandum from Daniel Nickerson, actuary, and Kyle Burkhalter, actuary, to Chris Chaplain, supervisory actuary, and Karen Glenn, deputy chief actuary, "Current-Law OASDI Payable Percentages: Current-Law Revenue as a Percent of the Cost of Providing Scheduled Benefits Through Year 2093—Information," May 20, 2019 (hereinafter "2019 OCACT Payable Benefits Memo").

Notes: Projections are based on the trustees' 2019 intermediate assumptions. In calculating the share of payable benefits, OCACT limits revenue from the taxation of benefits to the amount that would be obtained from the payable benefits.

Figure 3. Benefits as a Share of Scheduled Benefits, 2019-2093.

Replacement Rates

One way of measuring the adequacy of Social Security benefits is the *replacement rate*, the ratio of an individual's program benefit to past covered earnings. Replacement rates can be calculated in different ways. This chapter uses the following methodology employed by SSA's actuaries.[44]

---

[44] Under the Social Security program, the replacement rate for retired workers is the ratio of the Social Security benefit to the average of the highest 35 years of covered earnings, indexed to wage growth using the SSA's Average Wage Index (AWI). Other ways to measure replacement rates are discussed in Andrew G. Biggs and Glenn R. Springstead, "Alternate Measures of Replacement Rates for Social Security Benefits and Retirement Income," *Social Security Bulletin*, vol. 68, no. 2, October 2008, http://www.ssa.gov/policy/docs/ssb/v68n2/v68n2p1.html, and in SSA, OCACT, *Replacement Rates For Retirees: What Makes Sense For Planning And Evaluation?*, Actuarial Note 155, July 2014, at http://www.ssa.gov/oact/NOTES/pdf_notes/note155.pdf.

$$\text{Replacement Rate} = \frac{\text{Initial Social Security Benefit}}{\text{Career-Average Indexed Earnings from Covered Work}}$$

Social Security was established to replace income lost to a family as a result of the retirement, death, or disability of a worker. To ensure that average benefit levels grow along with average wages—thus keeping replacement rates generally steady—initial Social Security benefits are indexed to wage growth. Historically, wages have generally risen faster than prices, allowing the standard of living to rise from one generation to the next.

Figure 4 shows projected replacement rates under the benefit cut scenario for hypothetical low, medium, and high earners who claim retirement benefits at their full retirement age from 2019 through 2093.[45]

The Social Security benefit formula is progressive, so the replacement rate is higher for people with lower lifetime earnings in covered employment or self-employment than for people with higher lifetime earnings. In 2019, the estimated rates are 55% for low earners, 41% for medium earners, and 34% for high earners.[46]

Because lower earners have higher replacement rates, the 20% reduction would result in a larger *percentage point* reduction in replacement rates for low earners than for high earners. The replacement rate for low earners would fall from 55% in 2034 to 44% in 2035, a decline

[45] The low earner is assumed to have earned 45% of the national average wage (or $24,239 in 2019) when working and to receive an annual Social Security benefit of $13,243 in 2019. The medium earner is assumed to have earned the average wage (or $53,864 in 2019) and to receive a benefit of $21,843 in 2019. The high earner is assumed to have earned 160% of the average wage (or $86,182 in 2019) and to receive a benefit of about $28,934 in 2019. For more information, see 2019 Social Security Trustees Report, Table V.C7 (Supplemental Single-Year Tables) and SSA, OCACT, *Replacement Rates for Hypothetical Retired Workers*, Actuarial Note 2019.9, April 2019, Table C, https://www.ssa.gov/OACT/NOTES/ran9/an2019-9.pdf (hereinafter "OCACT Actuarial Note 2019.9"). For information on the development of the hypothetical workers, see SSA, OCACT, *Internal Rates of Return Under the OASDI Program for Hypothetical Workers*, Actuarial Note 144, June 2001, http://www.ssa.gov/oact/NOTES/note2000s/note144.html.

[46] OCACT Actuarial Note 2019.9, Table C.

of 11 percentage points. In contrast, the replacement rate for high earners would fall from 34% in 2034 to 27% in 2035, a 7-percentage-point drop.[47]

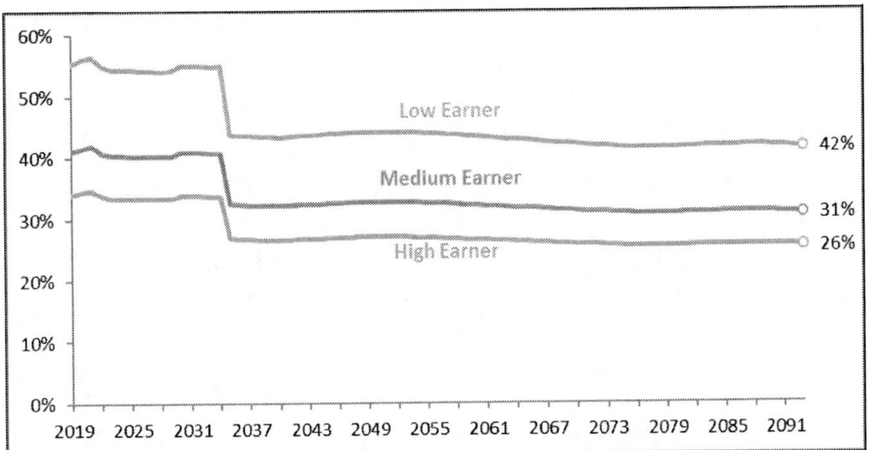

Source: CRS analysis of data from 2019 OCACT Payable Benefits Memo and SSA, OCACT, Replacement Rates for Hypothetical Retired Workers, Actuarial Note 2019.9, April 2019, Table C, https://www.ssa.gov/OACT/NOTES/ran9/an2019-9.pdf.

Notes: Projections are based on the trustees' 2019 intermediate assumptions. Replacement rates are for hypothetical earners who claim retirement benefits at their full retirement age.

Figure 4. Replacement Rates for Retired Workers Who Claim at Their Full Retirement Age Under the Benefit Cut Scenario, 2019-2093. (Initial benefits as a share of career-average indexed earnings from covered work)

Real Benefit Levels

Another measure of benefit adequacy is initial annual benefit amounts. Since benefits are based on workers' lifetime earnings, higher earners tend to receive higher benefit amounts than lower earners. In 2019, a hypothetical low earner is estimated to receive an annual Social Security benefit of $13,243, a medium earner a benefit of $21,843, and a high

[47] CRS analysis of data from OCACT Actuarial Note 2019.9, Table C, and OCACT memorandum from Daniel Nickerson, actuary, and Kyle Burkhalter, actuary, to Chris Chaplain, supervisory actuary, and Karen Glenn, deputy chief actuary, "Current-Law OASDI Payable Percentages: Current-Law Revenue as a Percent of the Cost of Providing Scheduled Benefits Through Year 2093—Information," May 20, 2019 (hereinafter "2019 OCACT Payable Benefits Memo").

earner a benefit of $28,934.[48] *Figure 5* shows future initial real benefit amounts in 2019 dollars (i.e., after adjusting for inflation), which illustrates how the purchasing power of benefits will change over time.

Because average real earnings generally grow over time, scheduled real benefits also grow. The trustees project that scheduled initial real benefit amounts for hypothetical individuals claiming retirement benefits at their full retirement age will increase by 25% between 2019 and 2035.[49] Under the benefit cut scenario, real payable benefit levels are projected to drop by 20% after the trust funds become insolvent in 2035, then to once again rise gradually.[50] Under the trustees' projections, payable benefits in 2035 would be about the same as payable benefits in 2019.[51]

Payroll Tax Increase Scenario

Upon trust fund depletion, the system could also be balanced by raising the payroll tax rate so that the tax income would be sufficient to pay scheduled benefits each year.

Size of Payroll Tax Rate Increases

The trustees project that paying scheduled benefits after depletion in 2035 would require an increase in the combined employee and employer payroll tax rate of 3.2 percentage points, from the current 12.4% to 15.6%, after insolvency in 2035.[52] To sustain balance, the payroll tax rate would have to reach 16.5% by 2093, the last year of the 75-year projection

---

[48] 2019 Social Security Trustees Report, Table V.C7 (Supplemental Single-Year Table). Benefits in 2019 dollars with retirement at full retirement age.

[49] Ibid.

[50] Immediately before the trust funds become insolvent in 2035, annual scheduled real benefits for individuals retiring at their full retirement age are projected to be $16,595 for the low earner, $27,366 for the medium earner, and $36,220 for the high earner. The annual payable real benefits would be 80% of these amounts. See 2019 Social Security Trustees Report, Table V.C7, (Supplemental Single-Year Table).

[51] CRS analysis of data from 2019 OCACT Payable Benefits Memo and 2019 Social Security Trustees Report, Table V.C7 (Supplemental Single-Year Table).

[52] CRS analysis of data from 2019 Social Security Trustees Report, Table IV.B1 (Supplemental Single-Year Table).

period.[53] *Figure 6* shows the combined payroll tax rate under current law and the combined payroll tax rate needed to pay scheduled benefits from 2019 to 2093.

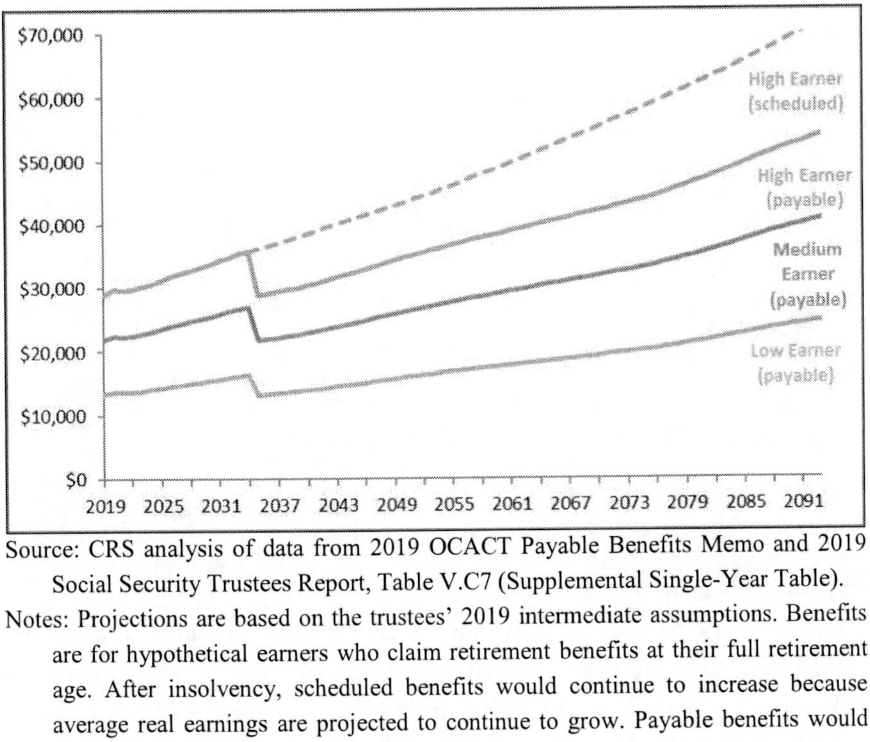

Source: CRS analysis of data from 2019 OCACT Payable Benefits Memo and 2019 Social Security Trustees Report, Table V.C7 (Supplemental Single-Year Table).

Notes: Projections are based on the trustees' 2019 intermediate assumptions. Benefits are for hypothetical earners who claim retirement benefits at their full retirement age. After insolvency, scheduled benefits would continue to increase because average real earnings are projected to continue to grow. Payable benefits would therefore also grow over time following the drop upon insolvency, though they would be permanently lower than scheduled benefits. For clarity, scheduled benefits are shown only for high earners.

Figure 5. Initial Real Annual Payable Benefits for Retired Workers Claiming at Their Full Retirement Age Under the Benefit Cut Scenario, 2019-2093. (in 2019 dollars)

---

[53] Ibid. Under the tax rate increase scenario discussed in this report, the payroll tax rate would have to change each year, increasing in some years and decreasing in others. Alternatively, the payroll tax rate could be permanently increased by 3.65 percentage points starting in 2035 (from 12.40% to 16.05%) to maintain solvency over the 75-year projection period. See footnote 42.

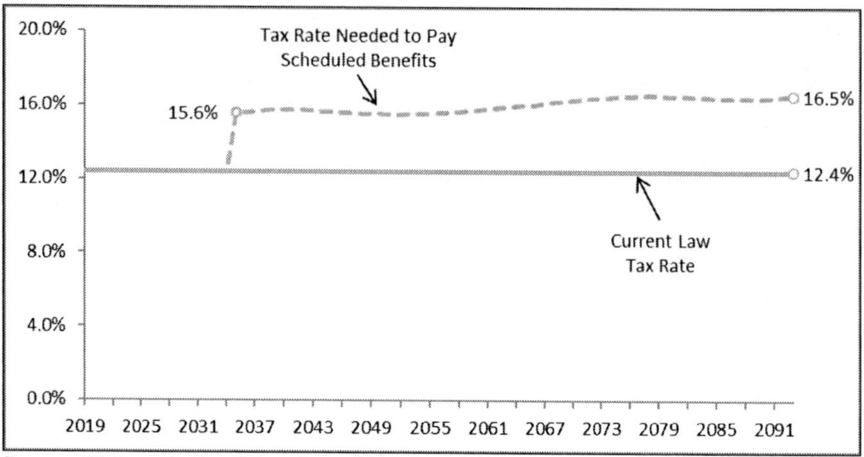

Source: CRS analysis of data from 2019 Social Security Trustees Report, Table IV.B1 (Supplemental Single-Year Table).

Notes: Projections are based on the trustees' 2019 intermediate assumptions. Under the trustees' projections, the current 12.4% combined payroll tax rate is sufficient to pay scheduled benefits prior to 2035 on a combined basis.

Figure 6. Combined Social Security Payroll Tax Rate Under Current Law and Under the Tax Rate Increase Scenario, 2019-2093.

Impact of Payroll Tax Increases

Raising the payroll tax rate would increase most workers' taxes by the same proportion. However, because covered earnings are taxable only up to a specified maximum ($132,900 in 2019), the effective increase in the payroll tax would be smaller in percentage terms for people who earn more than the taxable maximum than for other workers. Unlike the federal income tax, the Social Security payroll tax is levied at a flat rate starting at the first dollar of earnings.

CONCLUSION

Under current law, the Social Security trust funds will almost certainly become insolvent. The sooner changes are made to the program, the smaller and less abrupt the changes would need to be to maintain solvency. Prompt action would also allow Congress to gradually phase in changes, rather than abruptly cutting benefits or raising taxes, thus allowing workers to plan in advance for their retirements.

APPENDIX A. 2018 TRUST FUND OPERATIONS

Table A-1. Operations of the Social Security Trust Funds, 2018 (in millions of dollars)

Category	OASI Trust Fund	DI Trust Fund	Combined OASDI Trust Funds
Receipts			
Payroll and Self-Employment Taxes	$715,865	$169,186	$885,051
Income from the Taxation of Benefits	34,488	530	35,017
General Fund Reimbursements	18	3	22
Non-Interest Income	*$750,371*	*$169,719*	*$920,090*
Interest	80,655	2,628	83,283
Total	$831,026	$172,347	$1,003,373
Expenditures			
Benefit Payments	844,895	143,741	988,635
Administrative Expenses	3,800	2,856	6,656
Railroad Retirement Transfers	4,769	174	4,942
Total	$853,464	$146,770	$1,000,233
Balance (Asset Reserves)			
Balance at the Start of the Year	2,820,309	71,480	2,891,789
Net Increase	-22,437	25,577	3,140
Balance at the End of the Year	$2,797,872	$97,057	$2,894,929
Cash Flow Surplus/Deficit (Net Increase in Balance Less Interest Income)	-$103,092	$22,949	-$80,143

Source: CRS, based on SSA, OCACT, "Financial Data for a Selected Time Period," https://www.ssa.gov/oact/ ProgData/allOps.html.

Notes: OASI = Old-Age and Survivors Insurance. DI = Disability Insurance. OASDI = Old-Age, Survivors, and Disability Insurance. The Combined OASDI Trust Fund values may not necessarily equal the sum of its rounded components.

Appendix B. Key Dates Projected for the Social Security Trust Funds

Table B-1. Key Dates Projected for the Social Security Trust Funds as Shown Under the Intermediate Assumptions in Trustees Reports **from 1983 to 2018**

Year of Report	**Year of Projected Depletion**			**Year That Total Cost First Exceeds Non-Interest Income[a]**			**Year That Total Cost First Exceeds Total Income[a]**		
	OASI	DI	OASDI	OASI	DI	OASDI	OASI	DI	OASDI
Intermediate II-B Projections[b]									
1983	[c]	[c]	[c]	[d]	[d]	2021	[d]	[d]	2047
1984	[c]	2050	c	2021	2012	2021	2045	2038	2044
1985	2050	2034	2049	2019	2010	2019	2032	2020	2032
1986	2054	2026	2051	2020	2009	2019	2035	2017	2033
1987	2055	2023	2051	2020	2008	2019	2036	2013	2033
1988	2050	2027	2048	2019	2009	2019	2033	2016	2032
1989	2049	2025	2046	2019	2009	2018	2032	2014	2030
1990	2046	2020	2043	2019	2008	2017	2030	2011	2028
Intermediate Projections									
1991	2045	2015	2041	2018	1998	2017	2030	2011	2028
1992	2042	1997	2036	2018	1992	2016	2028	1992	2024
1993	2044	1995	2036	2019	1993	2017	2030	1993	2025
1994	2036	1995	2029	2016	1994	2013	2024	1994	2019
1995	2031	2016[e]	2030	2014	2003[e]	2013	2021	2007[e]	2020
1996	2031	2015	2029	2014	2003	2012	2021	2007	2019
1997	2031	2015	2029	2014	2004	2012	2021	2007	2019
1998	2034	2019	2032	2015	2006	2013	2023	2009	2021
1999	2036	2020	2034	2015	2006	2014	2024	2009	2022
2000	2039	2023	2037	2016	2007	2015	2026	2012	2025
2001	2040	2026	2038	2016	2008	2016	2027	2015	2027
2002	2043	2028	2041	2018	2009	2017	2028	2018	2027
2003	2044	2028	2042	2018	2008	2018	2030	2018	2028
2004	2044	2029	2042	2018	2008	2018	2029	2017	2028
2005	2043	2027	2041	2018	2005	2017	2028	2014	2027
2006	2042	2025	2040	2018	2005	2017	2028	2013	2027
2007	2042	2026	2041	2018	2005	2017	2028	2013	2027
2008	2042	2025	2041	2018	2005	2017	2028	2012	2027
2009	2039	2020	2037	2017	2005	2016	2025	2009	2024
2010	2040	2018	2037	2018	2005	2015	2026	2009	2025
2011	2038	2018	2036	2017	2005	2010	2025	2009	2023

Year of Report	Year of Projected Depletion			Year That Total Cost First Exceeds Non-Interest Income[a]			Year That Total Cost First Exceeds Total Income[a]		
	OASI	DI	OASDI	OASI	DI	OASDI	OASI	DI	OASDI
2012	2035	2016	2033	2010	2005	2010	2023	2009	2021
2013	2035	2016	2033	2010	2005	2010	2022	2009	2021
2014	2034	2016	2033	2010	2005	2010	2022	2009	2020
2015	2035	2016	2034	2010	2005	2010	2022	2009	2020
2016	2035	2023[f]	2034	2010	2019[f]	2010	2022	2019[f]	2020
2017	2035	2028	2034	2010	2019	2010	2022	2019	2022
2018	2034	2032	2034	2010	2019	2010	2020	2019	2018
2019	2034	2052	2035	2010	2036	2010	2020	2041	2020

Source: CRS, based on data from 1983-2019 Social Security Trustees Reports and information provided by SSA.

Notes: OASI = Old-Age and Survivors Insurance. DI = Disability Insurance. OASDI = Old-Age, Survivors, and Disability Insurance.

[a] Dates indicate the first year a condition is projected to occur and to persist annually thereafter through the end of the 75-year projection period.

[b] From 1983 to 1990, two intermediate forecasts were prepared (II-A and II-B). The intermediate II-B forecast corresponds more closely to the intermediate forecast in subsequent years.

[c] Trust fund expected to remain solvent throughout the long-range projection period.

[d] Not available.

[e] The Social Security Domestic Employment Reform Act of 1994 (P.L. 103-387) authorized a reallocation of the payroll tax rate between the OASI and DI trust funds to ultimately provide DI with more revenue.

[f] The Bipartisan Budget Act of 2015 (P.L. 114-74) authorized a temporary reallocation of the payroll tax rate between the OASI and DI trust funds to provide DI with more revenue for 2016 through 2018.

In: Key Congressional Reports for June 2019 ISBN: 978-1-53616-665-1
Editor: Amada A. Byrd

Chapter 7

THE RADIATION EXPOSURE COMPENSATION ACT (RECA): COMPENSATION RELATED TO EXPOSURE TO RADIATION FROM ATOMIC WEAPONS TESTING AND URANIUM MINING (UPDATED)*

Scott D. Szymendera

SUMMARY

The Radiation Exposure Compensation Act (RECA) provides one-time benefit payments to persons who may have developed cancer or other specified diseases after being exposed to radiation from atomic weapons testing or uranium mining, milling, or transporting. Administered by the Department of Justice (DOJ), RECA has awarded

* This is an edited, reformatted and augmented version of Congressional Research Service Publication No. R43956, Updated June 11, 2019.

over $2.3 billion in benefits to more than 35,000 claimants since its inception in 1990. The RECA program is scheduled to sunset in 2022.

RECA benefits are available to the following groups:

- onsite participants—$75,000 to persons who participated onsite in the atmospheric test of an atomic weapon and developed one of the types of cancers specified in the statute;
- downwinders—$50,000 to persons who were present in one of the specified areas near the Nevada Test Site during a period of atmospheric atomic weapons testing and developed one of the types of cancers specified in the statute; and
- uranium miners, millers, and ore transporters—$100,000 to persons who worked in mining, milling, or transportation of uranium between 1942 and 1971 and developed one of the types of diseases specified in the statute.

The RECA statute was last amended in 2000. Since then, Congress has frequently considered legislation to expand the downwinder-eligibility area by making persons who were affected in other states during periods of atmospheric atomic weapons testing eligible for benefits and by allowing uranium miners, millers, and ore transporters to qualify for benefits based on work after 1971. However, an expansion of the downwinder-eligibility area is not supported by a congressionally mandated National Research Council report on atomic test fallout, and the inclusion of post-1971 uranium work, which was largely for commercial rather than governmental purposes, is not consistent with the program's stated intent.

INTRODUCTION

The Radiation Exposure Compensation Act (RECA) was enacted in 1990 and provides one-time cash benefits to certain persons who participated in atomic weapons testing or lived near the Nevada Test Site during periods of atmospheric (above-ground) atomic weapons testing.[1] Benefits under RECA are also available to certain uranium miners, mill workers, and ore transporters who worked in the uranium industry between

[1] 42 U.S.C. §2210 note; enacted as P.L. 101-426 on October 15, 1990.

1942 and 1971, when the federal government stopped its procurement of uranium for the atomic weapons program. All RECA claimants must have contracted one of the medical conditions specified in the statute after possible exposure to ionizing radiation from the detonation of an atomic weapon or after working in the uranium industry.

The RECA program is administered by the Civil Division of the Department of Justice (DOJ).[2] To date, DOJ has approved more than 35,000 RECA claims for more than $2.3 billion in benefits. The majority of RECA claims are related to atomic weapons testing rather than the uranium industry. Complete RECA program data are provided in *Table A-1* in the *Appendix*.

Benefits under RECA are paid out of general revenue and are considered mandatory spending. Pursuant to the Radiation Exposure Compensation Act Amendments of 2000, P.L. 106-245, all RECA benefit applications must be filed before July 10, 2022, at which point the program is scheduled to sunset.[3]

ATOMIC WEAPONS TESTING AT THE NEVADA TEST SITE

On July 16, 1945, the United States detonated the first atomic bomb at the Trinity Test Site near Alamogordo, NM. This atomic weapons test, which was followed by the only two offensive uses of atomic weapons at Hiroshima and Nagasaki, Japan, ushered in an era of extensive development and testing of atomic weapons that would last until 1992. During this period, the United States, under the auspices of the Atomic Energy Commission (AEC) and later Department of Energy (DOE), conducted 1,054 atomic weapons tests.[4] The majority (928) of these tests were conducted at the Nevada Test Site (NTS), a 1,375 square-mile federal

---

[2] The Radiation Exposure Compensation Act (RECA) program website is at http://www.justice.gov/civil/common/reca. Implementing regulations are at Part 79 of Title 28 of the Code of Federal Regulations (C.F.R.).

[3] Section 8(a) of RECA, as amended by P.L. 106-245 provides a filing deadline that is 22 years after the date of enactment of the 2000 amendments (July 10, 2000).

[4] Twenty-four of these tests were jointly conducted with the United Kingdom.

reservation located approximately 65 miles north of Las Vegas in Nye County, Nevada.[5] Of the 928 tests conducted at NTS, 828 were underground tests and 100 were atmospheric tests in which the atomic weapons exploded at or above ground level, resulting in radioactive material being released into the atmosphere.[6] These 100 atmospheric tests and the initial Trinity test were the only atmospheric atomic weapons tests conducted in the continental United States and Alaska. *Table 1* provides a summary of U.S. atomic weapons tests by location.

Table 1. United States atomic weapons tests, by location

Location	Number of Tests
South Atlantic Ocean Area	3
Pacific Ocean Area	106
United States other than Nevada Test Site (NTS)	17
Alamogordo, NM (Trinity Test Site)	1
Amchitka, AK	3
Carlsbad, NM	1
Central NV	1
Fallon, NV	1
Farmington, NM	1
Grand Valley, CO	1
Hattiesburg, MS	2
Nellis Air Force Range, NV	5
Rifle, CO	1
NTS	928
Total	1, 054

Source: Department of Energy, United States Nuclear Tests: July 1945 through September 1992, DOE/NV-209-REV 15, December 2000, p. xiii.

Note: Includes 24 joint U.S.-U.K. tests conducted at NTS.

Atmospheric atomic weapons tests at NTS were conducted between January 27, 1951, and October 30, 1958, and again between July 7, 1962,

[5] The Nevada Test Site (NTS) is now referred to as the Nevada National Security Site and is administered by the Department of Energy (DOE), National Nuclear Security Administration. For additional information on the history and characteristics of the NTS, see Terrance R. Fehner and F.G. Gosling, *Origins of the Nevada Test Site*, Department of Energy, DOE/MA-0518, December 2000.

[6] During some underground tests, radioactive material escaped from underground through a process known as venting, thus releasing some radioactive material into the atmosphere.

and July 17, 1962. The largest atmospheric test at NTS in terms of energy yield was the Hood Test conducted on July 5, 1957, which had an energy yield equivalent to 74,000 tons (74 kilotons or kt) of trinitrotoluene (TNT).[7]

RECA BENEFITS

Compensation Payments

The following benefits are available under the RECA program:

- $75,000—*Onsite participants* (persons who were present at a test site during an atmospheric atomic weapons test);
- $50,000—*Downwinders* (persons who were present in certain areas north and west of NTS[8] during periods of atmospheric atomic weapons testing); and
- $100,000—*Uranium Workers* (uranium miners, uranium millers, and uranium ore transporters)

All benefits are one-time lump sum payments and are not adjusted to reflect changes in wages or the cost of living. Benefits are not subject to the federal income tax[9] but are offset by any payments received from any lawsuit or settlement, or by any disability compensation or Dependency and Indemnity Compensation (DIC) payments from the Department of Veterans Affairs (VA) for any illnesses or injuries due to exposure to radiation from atomic weapons testing or work in the uranium industry

---

[7] For comparison purposes, the first atomic bomb ever detonated had a yield of 21 kt; the atomic bombs dropped on Hiroshima and Nagasaki had yields of 15 kt and 21 kt, respectively; and the largest atmospheric test conducted by the United States, the Bravo Test at Bikini Atoll in the Marshall Islands on February 28, 1954, had a yield of 15 million tons (15 megatons or Mt).

[8] The areas eligible for downwinder compensation are listed in *Table 3* and provided in the map in the *Appendix*.

[9] 26 U.S.C. §104(a)(2).

covered by RECA.[10] For onsite participants with claims based on diseases other than leukemia, RECA benefits are offset by the actuarial present value of prior payments.[11] For all other beneficiaries, including onsite participants with claims based on leukemia with radiation exposure prior to age 21, RECA benefits are offset by the actual value of prior payments. A veteran who has received RECA benefits prior to the receipt of disability compensation benefits from the VA under the presumptive eligibility provisions of the Radiation-Exposed Veterans Compensation Act (REVCA)[12] is required to have his or her VA benefits reduced by the amount of his or her RECA benefits.[13]

No medical or other benefits are provided by the RECA program. However, uranium workers eligible for RECA are automatically eligible for an additional $50,000 in compensation and medical benefits that pay for all medical costs associated with their covered illnesses under Part B of the Energy Employees Occupational Illness Compensation Program Act (EEOICPA).[14]

Survivors' Benefits

Each onsite participant, downwinder, or uranium worker who qualifies for RECA is entitled to one benefit payment on his or her behalf. If the claimant is living, the benefit is paid to him or her directly. If the claimant

---

[10] Section 6(c)(2) of the Radiation Exposure Compensation Act (42 U.S.C. §2210 note).

[11] The actuarial present value of prior payments is calculated in accordance with 28 C.F.R. §79.75(e) and Appendix C to Part 79 of Title 28 of the C.F.R.

[12] P.L. 100-321. Under REVCA, certain conditions related to radiation exposure in veterans who were onsite participants; served during the American occupation of Hiroshima or Nagasaki, Japan; were interred as prisoners of war in Japan; or served in a capacity that would make them eligible membership in the Energy Employees Occupational Illness Compensation Program Act (EEOICPA) special exposure cohort (through work in the development of atomic weapons) are presumed to be service-connected for the purposes of eligibility for disability compensation benefits payable by the VA.

[13] 38 U.S.C. §1112(c)(4).

[14] 42 U.S.C. §7384u. Onsite participants and downwinders are not automatically eligible for the Energy Employees Occupational Illness Compensation Program Act (EEOICPA) and can only receive EEOICPA Part B benefits by establishing eligibility through work in the development, not testing, of atomic weapons.

is deceased, then the benefit is paid to the following survivors according to order of precedence:

1. spouse, provided the spouse was married to the claimant for at least one year before the claimant's death;
2. children, in equal shares;
3. parents, in equal shares;
4. grandchildren, in equal shares; and
5. grandparents, in equal shares.

Only the survivors listed above are eligible for RECA benefits, and if there are no such survivors to a claimant, no benefit is paid on that claim.

RECA ELIGIBILITY

Onsite Participants

To be eligible for RECA benefits, an onsite participant must meet exposure and disease requirements.

Exposure Requirements

A person may be eligible for RECA benefits if he or she was present onsite and participated in an atmospheric atomic weapons test conducted by the United States and meets the specific geographic and participation requirements provided in the RECA regulations.

Geographic Requirements

A person must have been within or above one of the following geographic areas during a period of atmospheric atomic weapons testing,[15] including for up to six months after the period of testing ended:

---

[15] The dates for each period of atmospheric atomic weapons testing are provided at 28 C.F.R. §79.31(d)(1).

- NTS;
- the Pacific Test Sites (Bikini Atoll, Enewetak Atoll, Johnston Island, Christmas Island, the test site for the shot during Operation Wigwam, the test site for Shot Yucca during Operation Hardtack I, and the test sites for Shot Frigate Bird and Shot Swordfish during Operation Dominic I) and the official zone around each site from which non-test affiliated ships were excluded for security and safety purposes;
- Trinity Test Site;
- the South Atlantic Test Site for Operation Argus and the official zone around the site from which non-test affiliated ships were excluded for security and safety purposes;
- any designated location within a naval shipyard, air force base, or other official government installation where ships, aircraft, or other equipment used in an atmospheric nuclear detonation were decontaminated; or
- any designated location used for the purpose of monitoring fallout from an atmospheric nuclear test conducted at NTS.[16]

Participation Requirements

A person must have held one of the following occupations and performed one of the following activities while onsite during a period of atmospheric atomic weapons testing, including for up to six months after the period of testing ended:

Required Occupations

- member of the Armed Forces;
- civilian employee or contract employee of the Manhattan Engineer District, the Armed Forces Special Weapons Project, the Defense Atomic Support Agency, the Defense Nuclear Agency, or the

[16] 28 C.F.R. §79.11(f).

Department of Defense or its components or agencies or predecessor components or agencies;

- employee or contract employee of the AEC, the Energy Research and Development Administration, or the Department of Energy;
- member of the Federal Civil Defense Administration or the Office of Civil and Defense Mobilization; or
- member of the U.S. Public Health Service;[17] and

Required Activities

- performed duties within the identified operational area around each atmospheric detonation of a nuclear device;
- participated in the decontamination of any ships, planes, or equipment used during the atmospheric detonation of a nuclear device;
- performed duties as a cloud tracker or cloud sampler;
- served as a member of the garrison or maintenance forces on the atoll of Enewetak between June 21, 1951, and July 1, 1952; between August 7, 1956, and August 7, 1957; or between November 1, 1958, and April 30, 1959; or
- performed duties as a member of a mobile radiological safety team monitoring the pattern of fallout from an atmospheric detonation of a nuclear device.[18]

Disease Requirements

An onsite participant must have contracted one of the types of cancers listed in *Table 2* after exposure to ionizing radiation from his or her participation in an atmospheric atomic weapons test.

---

[17] 28 C.F.R. §79.11(g)(1).
[18] 28 C.F.R. §79.11(g)(2).

Downwinders

To be eligible for RECA benefits as a downwinder, a person must meet specified exposure and disease requirements based on his or her physical presence near NTS, rather than through his or her participation in an atomic weapons test.

Exposure Requirements

A downwinder must have been physically present for a period of at least 24 consecutive months between January 21, 1951, and October 31, 1958; or for the entire period between June 30, 1962, and July 31, 1962, in one of the counties or geographic areas listed in *Table 3* and provided in the map in the *Appendix.*

Table 2. Specified cancers for eligibility as onsite participants and downwinders(all cancers must be primary cancers)

Onset of the disease was at least two years after first exposure to fallout		
Leukemia (other than chronic lymphocytic leukemia if exposure to fallout was after age 20)		
Onset of the disease was at least five years after first exposure to fallout		
Multiple Myeloma	Lymphomas (other than Hodgkin's disease)	Bile Duct Cancer
Brain Cancer	Breast Cancer (male or female)	Colon Cancer
Esophageal Cancer	Gall Bladder Cancer	Liver Cancer (except if cirrhosis or hepatitis B is indicated)
Ovarian Cancer	Pancreatic Cancer	Pharynx Cancer
Salivary Gland Cancer	Small Intestine Cancer	Stomach Cancer
Thyroid Cancer	Urinary Bladder Cancer	Lung Cancer

Source: 42 U.S.C. §2210 note.

Disease Requirements

A downwinder must have contracted one of the types of cancers listed in *Table 2* after exposure to ionizing radiation from an atmospheric atomic weapons test at NTS.

Table 3. Downwinder Eligibility Areas

Arizona	Nevada	Utah
Apache County	Eureka County	Beaver County
Coconino County	Lander County	Garfield County
Gila County	Lincoln County	Iron County
Navajo County	Nye County	Kane County
Yavapai County	White Pine County	Millard County
Mohave County north of the Grand Canyon	Clark County townships 13 through 16 at ranges 63 through 71	Paiute County San Juan County Sevier County Washington County Wayne County

Source: 42 U.S.C. §2210 note.

Uranium Workers Miners

To qualify for RECA benefits, a uranium miner must meet specific exposure and disease requirements.

Exposure Requirements

A uranium miner must have worked in an above-ground or underground uranium mine for at least one year during the period between January 1, 1942, and December 31, 1971, or must have been exposed to at least 40 working-level months (WLM) of radiation during this period, in one of the states listed in *Table 4*.[19]

A WLM is defined in the RECA statute as one working level of radiation exposure every work day for a month, or an equivalent exposure over a greater or lesser period of time. One working level of radiation exposure is defined as the concentration of decay products of radon that

19 Any state may apply for uranium worker eligibility state status. If determined by the Department of Justice (DOJ) that a uranium mine was operating in the state at any time during the period from January 1, 1942, to December 31, 1971, that state will be added to the list. However, no state has ever been added to the list of eligible states.

will release 130,000 megaelectron volts (MeV) of alpha energy per liter of air.[20]

Table 4. Uranium worker eligibility states

Arizona	Colorado	Idaho	New Mexico
North Dakota	Oregon	South Dakota	Texas
Utah	Washington	Wyoming	

Source: 42 U.S.C. §2210 note.

Notes: Any additional state may apply for inclusion in this list and will be included if it is determined by DOJ that a uranium mine was operating in the state at any time during the period from January 1, 1942, to December 31, 1971. No state has ever been added to the list of eligible states through this process.

Disease Requirements

A uranium miner must have developed lung cancer or one of the following nonmalignant respiratory diseases after exposure to radiation:

- fibrosis of the lung;
- pulmonary fibrosis;
- corpulmonale related to fibrosis of the lung;
- silicosis; or
- pneumoconiosis.

Millers and Ore Transporters

Uranium millers and ore transporters may qualify for RECA benefits if they meet specific exposure and disease requirements.

Exposure Requirements

A uranium miller must have been employed in a uranium mill in one of the states listed in *Table 4* for at least one year during the period from January 1, 1941, to December 31, 1971.

---

[20] Radiation exposure in mines is largely caused by the inhalation of radon gas and the short-lived solid decay products of radon. In the RECA statute, these decay products are referred to as "short half-life daughters of radon."

An ore transporter must have worked transporting uranium ore or vanadium-uranium ore from a uranium mine or mill in one of the states listed in *Table 4* for at least one year during the period from January 1, 1941, to December 31, 1971.

Disease Requirements

A uranium miller or ore transporter must have developed one of the following conditions after exposure to radiation:

- primary lung cancer;
- primary renal cancer;
- a chronic renal disease, such as nephritis or kidney tubal tissue injury; or
- a nonmalignant respiratory disease, specifically
  - fibrosis of the lung;
  - pulmonary fibrosis;
  - corpulmonale related to fibrosis of the lung;
  - silicosis; or
  - pneumoconiosis.

APPLICATION AND APPEALS PROCESS

Application Process

DOJ's Civil Division administers the RECA program and makes eligibility decisions on claims. Benefit claims must be submitted in writing and on standard application forms provided by DOJ.

The RECA statute requires that claimants submit "written documentation" of their illnesses to qualify for benefits, and the RECA regulations provide detailed requirements on the types of documents that must be submitted. Section 6(d)(5) of the RECA statute requires that in cases submitted by Native Americans, the application and payment procedures established by DOJ must "take into consideration and incorporate, to the fullest extent feasible, Native American law, tradition, and custom."

Application decisions for RECA benefits are made by an assistant director within the Constitutional and Specialized Torts Section, Torts Branch, of the DOJ Civil Division. Decisions must be made within 12 months of the receipt of a completed application and all supporting materials. If no decision is made within 12 months, the application is automatically approved for benefits.

Radiation Exposure Screening and Education Program

Section 4 of the 2000 RECA amendments authorized the Department of Health and Human Services (HHS) to provide grants to federal, state, and local health centers and nonprofit organizations to (1) conduct cancer screenings of persons who may be eligible for RECA and (2) provide assistance with securing the medical documentation needed to file RECA claims. These grants are administered by the HHS Health Resources and Services Administration (HRSA) as the Radiation Exposure Screening and Education Program (RESEP). There are currently eight RESEP clinics operating in Arizona, Colorado, New Mexico, Nevada, and Utah with one clinic providing services exclusively to Native Americans.[21] Applicants for RECA benefits are not required to be screened for cancer at RESEP clinics.

Appeals Process

An applicant who is denied RECA benefits may file an appeal with the DOJ, which is ruled on by an appeals officer appointed by the Assistant

[21] Additional information on the Radiation Exposure Screening and Education Program (RESEP) is available on the Department of Health and Human Services (HHS) website at http://www.hrsa.gov/gethealthcare/conditions/radiationexposure/index.html.

Attorney General of the Civil Division of DOJ. Appeals must be made in writing within 60 days of the initial decision, and the appeals officer must make a decision to affirm or reverse the initial decision or remand the case back to the assistant director for further action. An applicant dissatisfied with the outcome of his or her appeal may seek judicial review in the U.S. District Court.

Attorney's Fees

Applicants for RECA benefits and applicants filing appeals of benefit denials may be represented in all matters related to the program by licensed attorneys. In addition, Native American claimants may be represented by nonattorney representatives of tribal organizations. These are the only nonattorneys authorized to represent RECA claimants. Nonattorney representatives may not charge fees for their representation. The RECA statute provides the following limitations on fees that may be collected by licensed attorneys who represent RECA claimants:

- for initial claims in which the attorney entered into a contract with the claimant on or after July 10, 2000, 2% of the benefits awarded;
- for initial claims in which the attorney entered into a contract with the claimant before July 10, 2000, 10% of the benefits awarded; and
- for the resubmission of previously denied claims, 10% of the benefits awarded.

In the case of an unsuccessful claim, an attorney may recover his or her costs associated with representing the claimant. Pursuant to a 2007 decision by the U.S. Court of Appeals and subsequent regulations, an attorney representing a successful claimant may recover his or her expenses associated with the claim in addition to the 2% or 10% fee.[22]

---

[22] Hackwell v. United States, 491 F.3d 1229 (10th Cir. 2007); and 28 C.F.R. §79.74(b).

OUTSTANDING ISSUES

Members of Congress have introduced legislation to expand the eligibility area for downwinders and provide benefits to uranium workers who may have been exposed to radiation after 1971. While there have been no statutory changes to the RECA program since 2000, these outstanding issues will likely ensure that RECA remains on the congressional agenda and may be part of any attempts to reauthorize RECA beyond its 2022 sunset date.

Expansion of the Downwinder Eligibility Area

Under current law, to qualify for RECA benefits as a downwinder, a person must have been present in one of the designated counties in Arizona, Nevada, or Utah during a period of atmospheric testing at NTS. Residents of other areas during testing, including some areas closer to NTS than the designated downwinder areas, areas near the Trinity test site in New Mexico, or residents of Guam who may have been affected by fallout from atomic weapons testing in the Pacific Ocean area, are not eligible for benefits, and new downwinder eligibility areas cannot be added to the program through regulation or executive action.

However, even before RECA became a federal program, residents of areas outside of the current downwinder eligibility area had expressed concern about the health effects of fallout from atomic weapons testing and attempted to gain compensation from the federal government through the civil courts.[23] The inability of downwinders to win civil judgments against either the federal government or atomic weapons testing contractors was one of the factors that led Congress to create the RECA program in 1990.[24]

---

[23] For additional information on the history of the downwinder movement, see A. Costadina Titus, *Bombs in the Backyard: Atomic Testing and American Politics* (Reno, NV: University of Nevada Press, 2001).

[24] Lawsuits against the federal government for damages related to atomic weapons testing were barred by the principle of sovereign immunity and the discretionary function exemption to the Federal Tort Claims Act (FTCA; see Allen v. United States, 816 F.2d 1417 (10th Cir.

Eligibility Areas in Early Legislation to Compensate Downwinders

The first bills to provide compensation to civilian downwinders affected by atmospheric testing at NTS were introduced during the 96th Congress in 1979. In the House of Representatives, H.R. 4766 would have made the United States liable for damages caused by atmospheric atomic testing at NTS to downwinders with cancer, onsite participants, and sheep herds damaged by atmospheric tests in 1953. Coverage under this bill would have been provided to downwinders with leukemia, thyroid cancer, bone cancer, or any other cancer that occurred more often in the affected area than would be expected as determined by the Secretary of Health, Education, and Welfare.

The affected area for downwinder eligibility in H.R. 4766 was a rectangular area around NTS from 112 degrees to 117.5 degrees longitude and from 36.5 degrees to 39 degrees latitude. In addition to areas in Nevada, Utah, and a small part of Inyo County, California, this area includes the northern portions of Mohave and Coconino Counties in Arizona, but does not extend south as far as the Colorado River. The boundaries as proposed by H.R. 4766 are provided in the map in the *Appendix*.

A companion Senate bill (S. 1865) also would have made the United States liable for damages to downwinders, onsite participants, and affected sheep herds as well as uranium miners. The bill would have created a federal advisory board with the authority to add to the list of specified cancers. The affected area for downwinder eligibility was expressed in terms of counties and other geographic features and included the following areas:

1987) and In re Consolidated United States Atmospheric Testing Litigation, 820 F.2d 982 (9th Cir. 1987)). Lawsuits against atomic weapons testing contractors were barred by Section 1631 of the Department of Defense Authorization Act of 1985 (P.L. 98-525; commonly known as the Warner Amendment), which made lawsuits under the FTCA (already barred) the sole remedy for injuries due to exposure to radiation from atomic weapons tests thus providing immunity to any contractors involved in the atomic testing program. For additional information on the FTCA, see CRS Report R45732, *The Federal Tort Claims Act (FTCA): A Legal Overview.*

- in Arizona, the area north of the Grand Canyon and west of the Colorado River;
- in Nevada, the counties of Eureka, Lander, Lincoln, Nye, and White Pine; and
- in Utah, the counties of Beaver, Carbon, Duchesne, Emery, Garfield, Grand, Iron, Kane, Juab, Millard, Piute, San Juan, Sanpete, Sevier, Uintah, Washington, and Wayne.

In addition, the bill would have given the Secretary of Health, Education, and Welfare the authority to add to the list of affected areas.

Eligibility Areas in the Original RECA Statute and the 2000 Amendments

The original RECA statute included a smaller downwinder eligibility area than is currently covered by the program. Initially, only residents of the following areas were covered by RECA:

- in Arizona, the area north of the Grand Canyon and west of the Colorado River;
- in Nevada, the counties of Eureka, Lander, Lincoln, Nye, and White Pine and Clark County townships 13 through 16 at ranges 63 through 71; and
- in Utah, the counties of Beaver, Garfield, Iron, Kane, Millard, Piute, and Sevier.

The current downwinder eligibility area was established with the enactment of the 2000 RECA amendments, which added geographical areas in Arizona and Utah and created the current area described in *Table 3*.[25]

[25] The 2000 RECA amendments inadvertently excluded the portion of Mohave County, Arizona, that is north of the Grand Canyon that had been included in the original RECA legislation. This portion of Mohave County was added back to the downwinder eligibility area by Section 11007 of the 21st Century Department of Justice Appropriations Authorization Act, P.L. 107-273.

The initial and current RECA downwinder eligibility areas are provided in the map in the *Appendix*.

Legislative Attempts to Expand the Downwinder Eligibility Area

Since the enactment of the 2000 RECA amendments, numerous bills have been introduced over multiple Congresses to expand the downwinder eligibility area. These bills would have expanded eligibility for NTS downwinders to persons who were living in Colorado, Idaho, Montana, and New Mexico as well as in the entire states of Arizona, Nevada, and Utah during periods of atmospheric atomic weapons testing at NTS. Additional legislation would have created downwinder eligibility for persons living in Guam during atomic weapons testing in the Pacific and for persons affected by fallout from the initial Trinity test in New Mexico.

National Research Council Review of the RECA Downwinder Eligibility Area

In 2002, in response to a congressional mandate contained in the House report to accompany the 2002 Supplemental Appropriations Act for Further Recovery From and Response to Terrorist Attacks on the United States (P.L. 107-206), HRSA asked the National Research Council (NRC) Board on Radiation Effects Research to study scientific evidence related to the health effects of radiation exposure and make recommendations to Congress, including whether the RECA downwinder area should be expanded.[26] The NRC issued its final report on this study in 2005.[27]

The NRC concluded that any decisions on additional eligibility for downwinders should not be made solely on the basis of geographic area. Thus, it advised against simply adding more downwind counties.

---

[26] U.S. Congress, House Committee on Appropriations, Making Supplemental Appropriations for Further Recovery From and Response to Terrorist Attacks on the United States for the Fiscal Year Ending September 30, 2002, and for Other Purposes, report to accompany H.R. 4775, 107th Cong., 2nd sess., May 20, 2002, H.Rept. 107-480, p. 38.

[27] National Research Council, *Assessment of the Scientific Information for the Radiation Exposure Screening and Education Program*, 2005.

Citing studies showing that NTS fallout covered the entire country and that people living far beyond the current downwinder eligibility area may have been exposed to higher amounts of radiation, the NRC recommended an alternative science-based approach to determining downwinder eligibility for RECA benefits.

Individuals' exposure to fallout depended on multiple factors, including where they lived, the amount of time they spent outdoors, and their consumption of milk. That last factor is especially significant because the most important pathway of exposure was the ingestion of Iodine 131 (^{131}I)[28] through the consumption of milk from cows and goats that ate contaminated vegetation.[29]

To be equitable, the NRC report recommended that the RECA program use a model of probability of causation to evaluate individual claims for benefits instead of basing downwinder eligibility solely on geography and a presumption of eligibility. Under this model, each applicant's individual absorbed dose of radionuclides would be estimated using geographic, demographic, and behavioral factors and every person in the country would be eligible to apply for benefits. This estimated dose would then be used to calculate, using established radio-epidemiology formulas developed by NCI, the probability that the individual's specific type of cancer was caused by his or her exposure to ionizing radiation. Congress would then have to set the threshold at which to award benefits or perhaps award varying levels of benefits based on a sliding scale of probabilities.

This model, which is similar to one of the methods used to determine eligibility for benefits under Part B of EEOICPA and for disability compensation provided by the VA, has never been part of the RECA program or its amendments to expand the downwinder area. No legislation

---

[28] Iodine 131 is a radioactive isotope of the element iodine.

[29] National Cancer Institute, Estimated Exposures and Thyroid Doses Received by the American People from Iodine-131 in Fallout Following Nevada Atmospheric Nuclear Bomb Tests, October 1997. Additional information on this study, including detailed county-level data and an online calculator to estimate ^{131}I doses, is available at http://www.cancer.gov/cancertopics/causes/i131.

has ever been introduced to convert RECA downwinder eligibility from a model based on geography to one based on the probability of causation.

In addition, in both the EEOICPA and veterans' programs, the probability of causation model has been largely supplanted by a presumption of eligibility model similar to that used in RECA.[30]

The presumptive eligibility model used by RECA may be favored by some advocates for compensation because the probability of causation model recommended by the NRC is likely to result in fewer successful claims. This is due to the generally low levels of radiation exposure from fallout and the fact that ionizing radiation is not an especially potent cancer-causing agent. In the executive summary to its report, the NRC states,

> The scientific evidence indicates that in most cases it is unlikely that exposure to radiation from fallout was a substantial contributing cause to developing cancer. Moreover, scientifically based changes that Congress may make in the eligibility criteria for compensation in response to this report are likely to result in few successful claims. The committee is aware that such conclusion may be disappointing, but they have been reached in accordance with the committee's charge to base its conclusions on the results of best available scientific information.[31]

Benefits for Post-1971 Uranium Workers

Under current law, RECA benefits for uranium miners, millers, and ore transporters are only available if the worker was exposed to radiation during uranium work before 1972.

---

[30] In the case of the Energy Employees Occupational Illness Compensation Program Act (EEOICPA), the majority of cases paid have come through the Special Exposure Cohort process rather than the dose reconstruction process. In the case of veterans, the Radiation Exposed Veterans Compensation Act (REVCA; P.L. 100-321) was enacted in 1988 to provide a presumption of eligibility model for disability compensation benefits.

[31] National Research Council, Assessment of the Scientific Information for the Radiation Exposure Screening and Education Program, 2005, p. 4.

In the original RECA legislation, the December 31, 1971, cutoff date for uranium worker eligibility was selected because the federal government's procurement of uranium for atomic weapons ended in 1971.

Beginning in 1964 with the enactment of the Private Ownership of Special Nuclear Materials Act, P.L. 88-489, private ownership of uranium for fuel for nuclear power plants has been legal, creating an additional market for mined and milled uranium and ensuring that mining, milling, and transporting of uranium continued after the cutoff date for RECA eligibility.

Since the enactment of the 2000 RECA amendments, legislation has been introduced in Congress to expand RECA eligibility to uranium workers who may have been exposed to radiation after 1971. Legislation has also been introduced to include uranium mine core drillers in the RECA program and to require research into the health effects of uranium tailing piles.

Advocates for extending RECA eligibility for uranium work after 1971 argue that despite improved safety regulations enacted since 1971, including the enactment in 1977 of the Mine Safety and Health Act, P.L. 91-173, uranium workers, especially miners, remain at elevated risk for radon-induced diseases.[32] For example, the current Mine Safety and Health Administration (MSHA) annual exposure limit for radiation of 4 WLM[33] is higher than the annual exposure limit of 1 WLM recommended by the National Institute for Occupational Safety and Health (NIOSH), meaning that current uranium miners can be exposed to higher than recommended levels of radon while still being in compliance with federal safety standards.[34]

---

[32] See, e.g., Gary E. Madsen and Susan E. Dawson, "Unfinished Business: Radiation Exposure Compensation Act (RECA) for Post-1971 U.S. Uranium Underground Miners," *Journal of Health and Social Policy*, vol. 19, no. 4 (2004), pp. 45-59.

[33] 30 C.F.R. §57.5038.

[34] National Institute for Occupational Safety and Health, *A Recommended Standard for Occupational Exposure to Radon Progeny in Underground Mines*, October 1987.

The RECA program's intent, as expressed in Section 2 of the statute, is to make "partial restitution" to persons who were affected by fallout from atomic weapons tests and uranium miners who were working in mines "that were providing uranium for the primary use and benefit of the nuclear weapons program of the United States Government," in recognition that the "lives and health of uranium miners and of individuals who were exposed to radiation were subjected to increased risk of injury and disease to serve the national security interests of the United States."

An expansion of RECA to cover post-1971 uranium activities would largely cover workers in the commercial uranium sector, which would expand the program beyond its original statutory intent. In addition, illnesses contracted during uranium mining, milling, and ore transporting for commercial clients, rather than the federal government, would likely be covered by existing state workers' compensation systems, which are the traditional means of providing medical benefits and compensation in cases of commercial workplace injuries, illnesses, or deaths.

APPENDIX. RECA PROGRAM DATA AND DOWNWINDER AREA MAP

Table A-1. RECA program claims data (as of June 3, 2019)

Claim Type	Pending	Approved	Denied	Total	Benefits Approved ($)
Onsite Participant	111	4,625	3,585	8,321	337,087,709
Downwinder	265	22,523	4,665	27,453	1,126,120,000
Uranium Miner	45	6,532	3,832	10,409	652,474,560
Uranium Miller	13	1,802	555	2,370	180,200,000
Ore Transporter	4	367	157	528	36,700,000
Total	438	35,849	12,794	49,081	2,332,582,268

Source: Department of Justice, Radiation Exposure Compensation System, Awards to Date Summary of Claims Received by 06/03/2019, June 4, 2019, https://www. justice.gov/civil/awards-date-06042019.

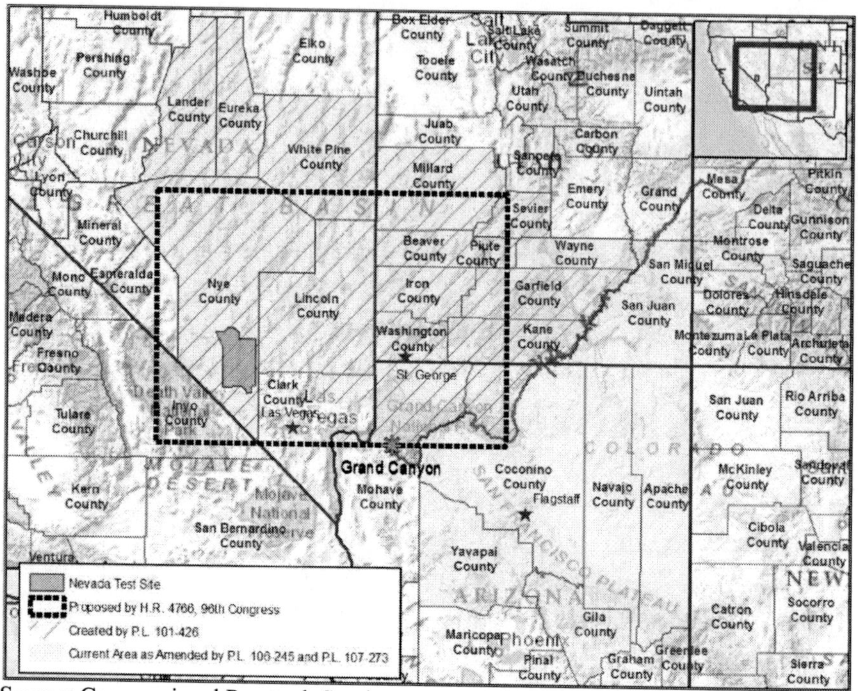

Source: Congressional Research Service.

Figure A-1. RECA Downwinder Area.

INDEX

#

A

B

C

D

E

P

R

S

T

U

W

Y

Related Nova Publications

Key Congressional Reports for February 2019. Part III

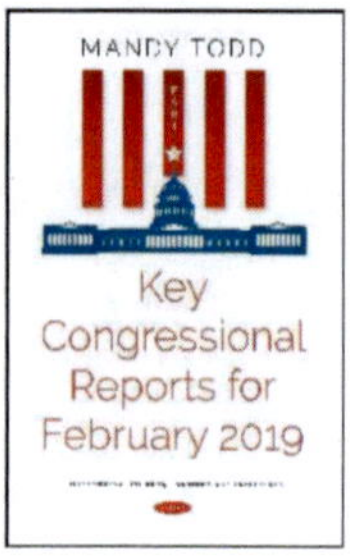

Editor: Mandy Todd

Series: Congressional Policies, Practices and Procedures

Book Description: This book is a comprehensive compilation of all reports, testimony, correspondence and other publications issued by the Congressional Research Service during the month of March, grouped according to topics.

Hardcover ISBN: 978-1-53615-997-4
Retail Price: $230

Key Congressional Reports for March 2019. Part I

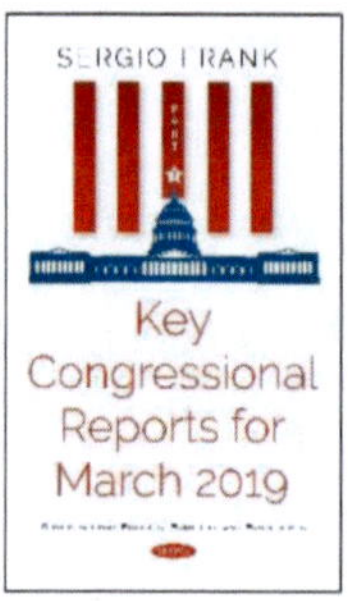

Editor: Sergio Frank

Series: Congressional Policies, Practices and Procedures

Book Description: This book is a comprehensive compilation of all reports, testimony, correspondence and other publications issued by the Congressional Research Service during the month of March, grouped according to topics. This book is focused on the following topics:
· Information Security & Technology
· Military Technology

Hardcover ISBN: 978-1-53615-976-9
Retail Price: $160